PHARMACOLOGY UNIVERSITY QUESTIONS FULLY SOLVED

HARI KRISHNA V S
MEDCARE BOOKS

Copyright © HARI KRISHNA V S, Medcare Books
All Rights Reserved.

This book has been self-published with all reasonable efforts taken to make the material error-free by the author. No part of this book shall be used, reproduced in any manner whatsoever without written permission from the author, except in the case of brief quotations embodied in critical articles and reviews.

The Author of this book is solely responsible and liable for its content including but not limited to the views, representations, descriptions, statements, information, opinions and references ["Content"]. The Content of this book shall not constitute or be construed or deemed to reflect the opinion or expression of the Publisher or Editor. Neither the Publisher nor Editor endorse or approve the Content of this book or guarantee the reliability, accuracy or completeness of the Content published herein and do not make any representations or warranties of any kind, express or implied, including but not limited to the implied warranties of merchantability, fitness for a particular purpose. The Publisher and Editor shall not be liable whatsoever for any errors, omissions, whether such errors or omissions result from negligence, accident, or any other cause or claims for loss or damages of any kind, including without limitation, indirect or consequential loss or damage arising out of use, inability to use, or about the reliability, accuracy or sufficiency of the information contained in this book.

Made with ♥ on the Notion Press Platform
www.notionpress.com

Contents

Preface   v

Acknowledgements   vii

1. General Pharmacology   1
2. Autonomous Nervous System   11
3. Skeletal Muscle Relaxants   23
4. Autacoids   25
5. Cardiovascular System   33
6. Respiratory System   46
7. Blood   51
8. Renal Pharmacology   54
9. Central Nervous System   58
10. Chemotherapy   76
11. Gastro Intestinal Drugs   104
12. Hormones And Related Drugs   112
13. Miscellaneous   129
14. Assertion And Reason Questions   135

Preface

Pharmacology, what makes pharmacology so special? It is a science of medical drug and medication, including a substance's origin, composition, pharmacokinetics, therapeutic use, and toxicology. In short, it is the study about the all the drugs which are going to be prescribed by us after becoming a doctor. So having a clear-cut idea about the drugs their uses its reactions with other drugs, its pharmacodynamics and pharmacokinetics are essential to become a good doctor. But the paradox is that even though it should be known top to bottom by every medical aspirant, it is a highly volatile subject. So that revising all the core topics of the pharmacology regularly from the starting of the second year MBBS holds a prime importance. The strategy that we have adopted to make the book concise is, including the answers of questions which is asked about a drug under the short note about the drug so as to make the content more concise as well as effective. Most of the questions that comes in university are repeating and we have put our effort to represent all those questions in this book without repetition. At the same time revising everything from the standard textbooks regularly is also not humanly possible. There comes the importance of this book, an endeavour by the 2019 batch students of the GMC Kolam. A book which consists of all the questions and answers of the previously asked questions in the KUHS which will make you able to revise the questions as fast as possible and also to obtain high scores.

    With love MedCareBooks

Acknowledgements

MedCareBooks

"MedCareBooks" is a group of medical students of 2019 Batch of Government medical college Kollam, who have pledged to make the medical education simpler as well as qualitative for others.

The main contributors of this book are

1. Hari Krishna V S (Chief editor)
2. Dr. Arun Anil
3. Dr. Nandu G
4. Dr. Happy K Premdas
5. Dr. Mythili M R
6. Dr. Mohammed Zakariya Hamza
7. Dr. Mirzed Mohammed M S

For feed backs suggestions write to us at medcarebooks@gmail.com

For getting 10% discount on all the courses and books at "medlive" app by Dr. Priyanka Sachdev MD use coupon code "QMCIANS"

For direct orders contact Whatsapp 9747792086

CHAPTER I

General Pharmacology

Routes of drug administration

1. Two advantages and disadvantages of iv route of drug administration?

    Ans)

Advantages	Disadvantages
1) Action of drug is faster	1) Preparation should be sterile
2) Can be used for drugs which are irritant	2) Preparations are expensive
3) Have high first pass metabolism, are destroyed by digestive enzymes	3) Need aseptic conditions
	4) Need skills for administration
	5) Can cause local injury to tissues nerves etc.

    Table : Advantages and disadvantages of i.v route

2. New drug delivery systems?

    Ans)

- Ocusert - Pilocarpine ocusert in glaucoma (Kept beneath lower eyelid - One week sustained release)
- Progestasert - Hormonal IUD of progesterone
- Liposomes - Helps in targeted drug delivery e.g., Liposoal infusion of Amphotericin B
- Monoclonal antibodies
- Drug-eluting stents
- Computerised miniature pumps E.G., Insulin pump

3. Advantages of inhalational sublingual routes of drug administration?

Ans) Rapid effect, Low dose is enough so that systemic toxicity can be reduced, Low first pass metabolism and high bioavailability.

4. Trans dermal drug delivery system?

Ans) It is a controlled drug delivery system given as a patch/ ointment, releases drug through the skin to the systemic circulation at a constant rate.

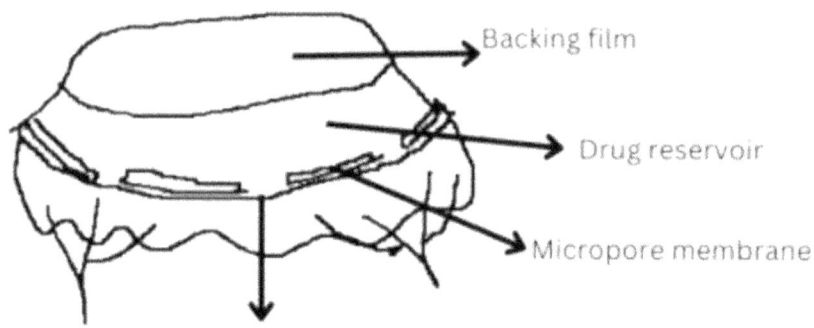

Img : Transdermal patch

Advantages	Disadvantages
Doesn't need to remember to take the drug	Expensive
Maintains a constant drug level in the blood	Can fell off from the body un-noticed
Can stop the action of the drug by taking off the patch	Skin irritation can cause at the place of the patch

Table : Uses and disadvantage of transdermal patch

Examples: Scopolamine patch for motion sickness, Clonidine patch for hypertension

5. Name two orphan drugs?

Ans) Ivacaftor, Alglucerase

Pharmacokinetics

The difference between pharmacokinetics and pharmacodynamics is that the former is what our body does to the drug and the latter is what the drug does to the body. Remember by the rhyme "drug does dynamics".

1. Bio availability of a drug?

   Ans) Bioavailability of a drug is the proportion of the drug which became available in the systemic circulation to the amount of the drug that consumed. So, the drugs administered through the intravenous route have the highest bioavailability, i.e., 100% by definition and is generally followed by intra muscular route and the oral route have the least bio availability. Factors affecting bioavailability - First pass metabolism, Hepatic diseases, Entero hepatic recycling.

2. First pass metabolism?

   Ans) First pass metabolism or pre-systemic metabolism is the metabolism a drug undergoes before reaching the systemic circulation. The drugs which are taken orally are undergoing highest first pass metabolism and the drugs taken intra venously the lowest. Drugs with high first pass metabolism have the lowest bioavailability and vice versa.
   Effects
   • Some drugs which are of high first pass metabolism is not effective orally. E.g., Isoprenaline, Lidocaine, Testosterone, Hydrocortisone
   • Some drugs with high first pass metabolism require higher doses for getting their effect. E.g., Propranolol, Salbutamol, Glyceryl trinitrate
   • Drugs with low first pass metabolism may cause toxicity even at lower doses. E.g., Theophylline

3. Apparent volume of distribution?

   Ans) It is the apparent volume of the drug is distributed assuming that the drug is distributed uniformly all over the body. Some drugs concentrate more in the tissues so that the concentration of the drug in the blood will be less for example digoxin and propranolol. For lipid insoluble drugs which do not enter the cells the volume of distribution will be same as that of the extra cellular fluid volume e.g., Gentamycin, Streptomycin etc. High plasma protein binding means high volume of distribution for example Aprepitant.

The factors which governs the volume of distribution of a drug is

- Lipid:Water partition coefficient ratio (As it increases Vd also increases)
- Plasma protein binding decreases free fraction and the volume of distribution
- Congestive cardiac failure Vd decreases

4. Plasma protein binding?

Ans) Protein bound drugs is not available for action. High plasma protein binding means high volume of distribution and long acting. e.g., Acidic and neutral drugs are generally bound to Albumin

5. Plasma half-life and its clinical significance?

Ans) Plasma half-life of a drug is defined as the time required for a drug to reach half of its initial concentration. For a drug there are 2 types of half-lives. Distributary half-life and eliminatory half-life. Initially when a drug is administered it gets distributed rapidly over the body which gives a very small half-life called distributary half-life and after getting distributed all over the body the concentration of the drug in the body again decreases due to elimination of the drug which gives an eliminatory half-life. The eliminatory half-life of the drug is called half-life of the drug.

Clinical significance: It is helpful for determining the excretion rates as well as steady-state concentrations for any specific drug. Nearly complete elimination of the drug takes place after 4 to 5 half-lives. For drugs eliminated by first order kinetics half-life remains constant because volume and clearance do not change with dose. For zero order kinetics, t½ increases with dose because clearance progressively decreases as dose is increased.

5. Microsomal enzyme induction?

Ans) Microsomes located in the smooth endoplasmic reticulum of liver cells release microsomal enzymes. Its release can be enhanced by certain drugs and environmental pollutants which will cause the increased biotransformation of the inducing drug itself or other drugs which are metabolised by these microsomal enzymes. 2 types selective (e.g., DDT) and nonselective (e. g., Phenobarbitone)

Clinically relevant examples

- Rifampicin treatment for the ones who are on oral contraceptives causes OCP failure.
- Administration of phenobarbitone for neonatal jaundice.
- Use of antiepileptics for long-term can cause osteomalacia
- In chronic smokers and alcoholics due to the presence of some enzymes induced due to it causes failure of some enzymes which are metabolized by the same enzyme.
- Due to the autoinduction i.e., the drug causes production of an enzyme which increases the metabolism of the same drug can cause tolerance to the drug so that more dose of the same drug may be required to produce the required effect e.g., Carbamazepine

6. What is a prodrug? and mention it's 2 uses?

Ans) Prodrug is an inactive form of a drug which gets metabolized to the active derivative in the body.

Drug	Prodrug	Use
Dopamine	Levo-dopa	Since dopamine cannot cross blood brain barrier, Levodopa crosses the BBB and gets converted into dopamine to increase the concentration of the dopamine in the CNS
Ampicillin	Bacampicillin	Reduces the side effects of ampicillin due to its better absorption

Table : Drug prodrug uses and adr

7. Kinetics of elimination?

   Ans)

Zero order	First order
A constant amount of the drug is eliminated from the body in a unit time	The rate of drug absorption is directly proportional to its plasma concentration.
Half-life of the drug is not a constant	Half-life of the drug is a constant
e.g., Phenytoin and aspirin at high concentration when excretion of drug is saturated	e.g., Phenytoin and aspirin at low concentration when excretion of drug is not saturated

   Table : Kinetics of elimination

8. Hoffman elimination?

   Ans) In it the drug gets excreted in the plasma itself by changing the configuration of the drug e.g., Atracurium and cis-atracurium

   •••

Pharmacodynamics

1. G-protein coupled receptors?

   Ans) It is the largest family of integral proteins which are included in many physiological as well as pathological processes in our body. They are linked to the effector by one or more GTP linked protein.

   Function: They transduce the different signals mediated by different signaling molecules.

Mechanism: The G-protein have 3 subunits α, β and Ý subunits. In the inactive state the α subunit is bind to the GDP. Activation of receptor leads to its replacement with GTP and the detachment of α subunit from the other 2 subunits and causes either activation or inactivation of the effector

2. Physiological antagonism?

Ans) Exhibited by insulin and glucagon; Adrenaline and histamine. They are present in our body and act at different sites to give opposite actions

3. Drug antagonism?

Ans) One drug inhibits the action of other drug is called antagonism.
It can be chemical as of by chelating agents, Physiological as of by insulin and glucagon or receptor level as competitive, or noncompetitive antagonism.
Competitive antagonism: Also known as surmountable or reversible type of antagonism. The inhibitor competes with the substrate for the same site as that of the substrate. It is a reversible type of antagonism which means when large quantity of substrate is added the antagonism is reversed. Causes right ward parallel shift in the dos- response curve E.g.: Naloxone and morphine
Non-competitive antagonism: The antagonist binds to site other than the active site called allosteric site which causes conformational changes to the enzyme so that the substrate can't bind to the enzyme. It is an irreversible type of antagonism which means when large quantity of substrate is added the antagonism is not reversed. Causes flattening of dose-response curve.

4. Chemical antagonism with one example?

Ans) Two chemicals react antagonistically to neutralize the effect e.g., Antacids neutralizes the hydrochloric acid in the treatment of peptic ulcer, Deferoxamine in the treatment of chronic iron overload.

5. What is a receptor? And discuss the various transducer mechanisms by which receptors act?

Ans) Receptor is a class of cellular macromolecules which are concerned specifically and directly with chemical signals between and within cells.

- G-protein coupled receptors (Discussed earlier)
- Ion channel receptor.

Also called ligand gated ion channels encloses specific channels for specific ions like Na+, K+ etc. e.g., Nicotinic receptors, GABAA receptor etc.

- Transmembrane enzyme-linked receptors

In which the binding of an extracellular ligand causes enzymatic activity on the intracellular side. e.g., Epidermal growth factor receptor, Glial cell derived neurotropic factor receptor etc.

Transmembrane JAK-STAT binding receptors

- cytokines bind to transmembrane receptors
- receptor associated JAKs are activated
- JAKs phosphorylates STAT proteins
- forms homo or heterodimer
- transferred to the nucleus
- regulates gene transcription

8. Receptors regulating gene expression.

Also called as nuclear receptors which are activated by lipid-soluble signals that can cross the plasma membrane like steroid hormones.

• • •

Pharmacotherapy

1. Tachyphylaxis with examples?

Ans) Tachyphylaxis also known as acute tolerance. In which tolerance to a drug develops rapidly which reduces the effect of the drug. E.g., Ephedrine, Nicotine

2. Therapeutic window phenomenon?

Ans) It is a phenomenon shown by some drugs in which the therapeutic dose range is very narrow below which the drug gives sub therapeutic effects above which it becomes toxic. E.g., Digoxin, Digitoxin

3. Young's formula?

Ans) For dose calculation of children

$$\text{Child dose} = \left(\frac{Age}{Age+12}\right) * Adult\ dose$$

Formula 1

• • •

Adverse drug reactions

1. Idiosyncrasy?

Ans) It is the abnormal activity of a specific drug to a specific individual. Can be exaggerated or lack of response. e.g., Chloramphenicol producing aplastic anaemia, Atypical pseudocholinesterase resulting in succinylcholine apnea.

2. Pharmacovigilance?

Ans) Science and activities relating to the detection, assessment, understanding and prevention of adverse effects or any other drug related problems (definition by WHO).

3. Pharmacogenetics and pharmacogenomics?

Ans) Pharmacogenetics is the study of how an individual's genetic variations affect their response to specific drugs whereas in pharmacogenomics an individual's whole genetic makeup to predict their response to drugs across multiple therapeutic areas.

4. Teratogenicity?

Ans) It is the capacity of a drug to cause abnormalities in the foetus when taken by mother. E.g., Thalidomide which causes phocomelia, Carbamazepine which causes neural tube defects, Valproate sodium which causes spina bifida

CHAPTER II

Autonomous nervous system

Cholinergic system

1. Explain briefly why physostigmine is preferred over neostigmine for the treatment of glaucoma?

    Ans) Physostigmine is a tertiary amine which absorbs through eye where are being a quaternary amine neostigmine doesn't

2. Treatment of smoking cessation?

    Ans) First line treatment includes Nicotine replacement therapy which works by progressively reducing the nicotine uptake by the patient. Bupropion which inhibits the noradrenaline and dopamine reuptake is also used.

3. Atropine as an antisecretory agent?

    Ans) Since atropine reduces all secretions it can act as an antisecretory agent. Due to the blockade of the M3 receptors it reduces the secretions of sweat, salivary gland, nasal etc. It makes the skin and mucous membrane dry

4. Therapeutic uses and adverse effects of atropine?

    Ans) <u>Uses</u>

- For organophosphate poisoning
- For COPD and bronchial asthma
- Mushroom poisoning by Inocybe species

- Dysmenorrhoea, Intestinal and renal colic
- Refraction testing, Fundoscopic examination, Iridocyclitis
- As preanaesthetic medication

<u>Adverse effects</u>

- Tachy cardia, Palpitation and hypotension
- Photophobia, Headache, Blurring of vision, Miosis
- Dry mouth, Difficulty in swallowing, Constipation
- Difficulty in micturition

5. Rationale for use of physostigmine in atropine poisoning?

   Ans) The physostigmine inhibits the acetylcholinesterase by inhibiting it synaptic acetyl choline break down is decreased and increases its concentration. Since it is a tertiary amine and can cross the blood-brain barrier it can reduce the central effects of atropine poisoning also

6. Explain the rationale for the use of oximes in organophosphorus poisoning (Anticholinesterase poisoning)?

   Ans) Oximes bind to the anion binding site of the acetyl choline esterase enzyme and makes it free by releasing the enzyme making bond between oximes and organophosphorus

7. Enumerate the topical group of agents used in the treatment of open angle glaucoma with mechanism?

   Ans)

Group of drugs	Examples	Mechanism of action
Miotics	Pilocarpine	Facilitates the drainage of aqueous humour
Carbonic anhydrase inhibitors	Acetazolamide Dorzolamide Brinzolamide	Decreases the formation of aqueous humour
Alpha-adrenergic agonists	Apraclonidine, Dipivefrine	Decreases the formation of aqueous humour
Beta blockers	Timolol, Carteolol, Betaxolol, Levobunolol	Decreases the formation of aqueous humour
Prostaglandins	Latanoprost, Bimatoprost, Travoprost	Facilitates uveoscleral outflow

8. Atropine or phenylnephrine used for refraction testing?

Ans) Atropine is the preferred choice for refraction testing due to its additional effect of paralyzing the ciliary muscle, which helps in obtaining accurate measurements.

9. Mention four atropine substitutes and the clinical indications for the same?

Ans) Scopolamine - Used primarily for motion sickness and postoperative nausea and vomiting

Glycopyrrolate - Used to reduce salivation and bronchial secretions during surgery, and to treat peptic ulcers

Ipratropium - Used as a bronchodilator in the management of chronic obstructive pulmonary disease (COPD) and asthma

Tropicamide - Used as a mydriatic and cycloplegic agent in ophthalmology for diagnostic purposes

Hyoscyamine - Used to treat gastrointestinal disorders such as irritable bowel syndrome (IBS) and colic

10. Physostigmine?

Ans) Physostigmine is used in atropine poisoning and glaucoma. Glaucoma it is used because of its good penetrating power in eye than Neostigmine.

11. Why atropine is given preoperatively? What are the other drugs which can be given preoperatively?

Ans) It is to reduce mucous secretions such as saliva. Reduces bronchial secretions there by reduces the chances of aspiration pneumonia.
Other drugs - Propofol, Fentanyl, Midazolam, Inhaled fluorinated ethers such as sevoflurane and desflurane.

12. Management of organophosphate poisoning?

Ans) <u>General measures</u>
Make the scene clear. Remove the clothes contaminated by organophosphate, Wash the body parts which were in contact with the organophosphate using soap and water. Maintain Airway, Breathing and Circulation (ABCs), Gastric lavage, Slow iv diazepam to control convulsions
Specific measures

- Atropine 2 mg i.v. stat, repeat every 5-10 minutes till the patient is fully atropinized. Continue atropine for 7-10 days
- Oximes for neuromuscular paralysis.

13. Name 2 vasicoselective anticholinergics?

Ans) Oxybutynin, Flavoxate

• • •

Adrenergic system

1. Prazosin?

Ans) Pharmacodynamics- It is a highly selective α1 blocker. All subtypes of α1 receptor (α1A, α1B, α1D) are blocked equally. Prazosin dilates arterioles more than veins.

Pharmacokinetics - Prazosin is effective orally, highly bound to plasma proteins (mainly to α1 acid glycoprotein), metabolized in liver and excreted primarily in bile.

Uses - As an antihypertensive, benign hypertrophy of prostate (BHP), Urinary retention and Raynaud's disease.

In the BHP it improves urinary flow rates by relaxing smooth muscles.

Adverse effects - It causes fall in BP. Which accounts for the first dose phenomenon. First dose phenomenon means in the beginning of the drug usage occurs fall in BP. To nullify this effect the drug is usually prescribed in the hour of sleep also by starting a lower dose in the beginning. It also causes dizziness and light headedness.

2. Classification of Alpha blockers?

Ans)

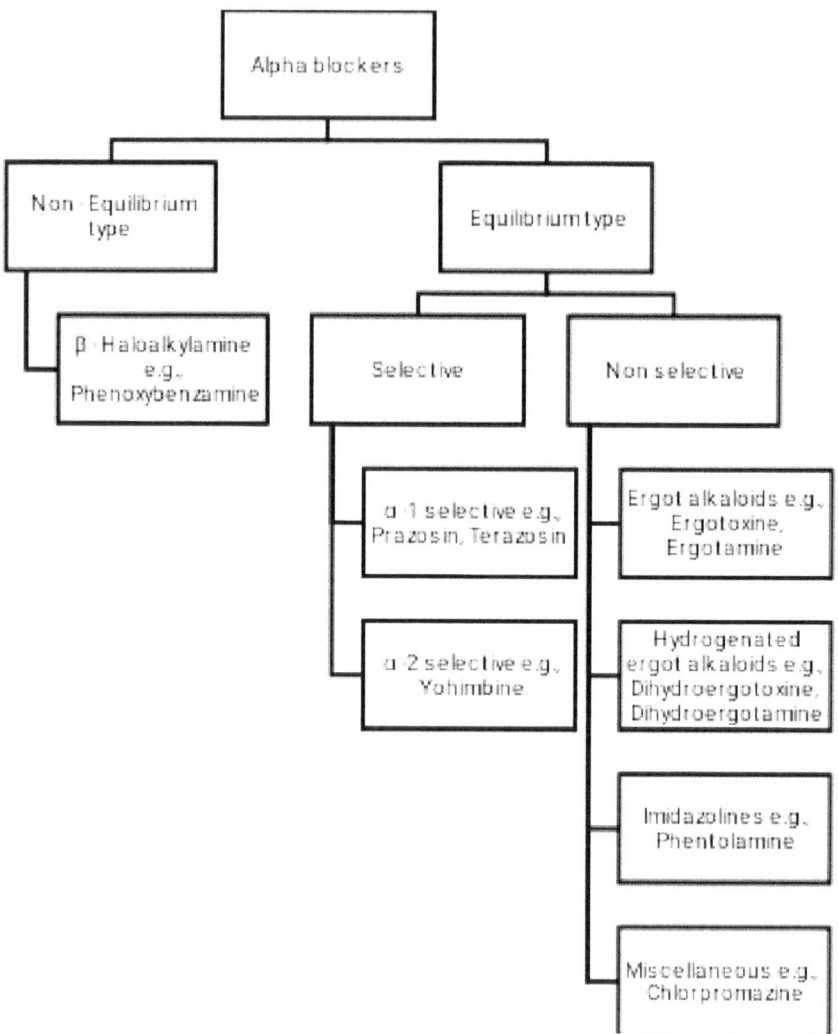

Enter Caption

3. Classification of Beta blockers?

   Ans) Generation wise classification

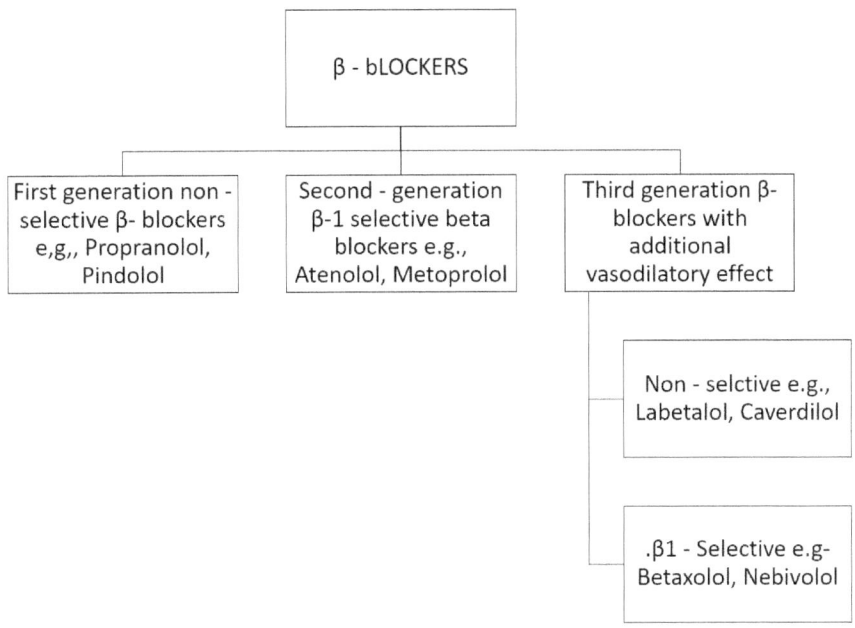

Classification according to receptor selectivity

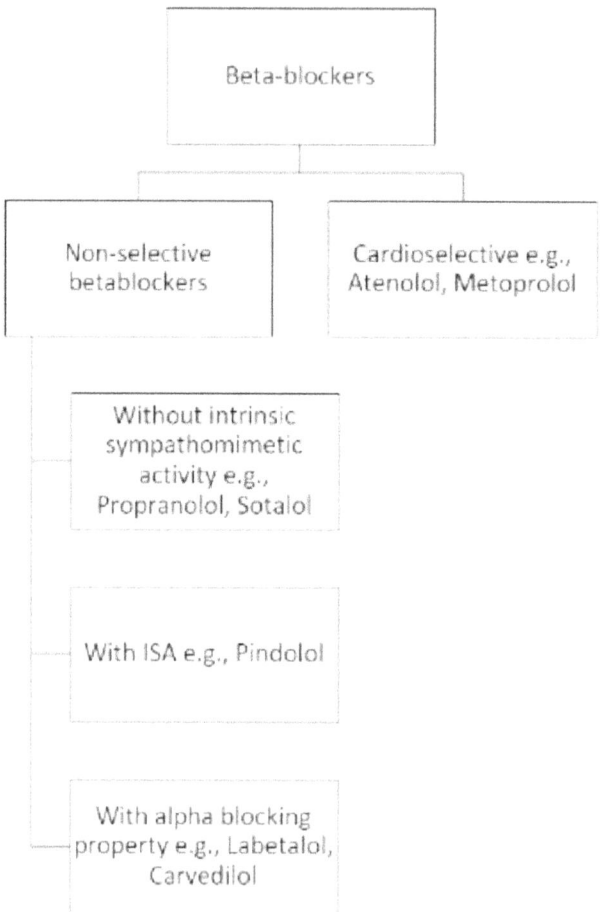

4. Propranolol uses and adverse effects?

Ans) Uses: To treat high blood pressure, Thyrotoxicosis, tremors and atrial fibrillation.

Adverse effects: Heart failure, feeling dizzy or tired, Cold hands or feet, Difficulties in sleeping and night mares.

5. Dipivefrine?

Ans) It is a prodrug of epinephrine used for the treatment of glaucoma. Uses – To treat chronic open angle glaucoma, and ocular hypertension. Adverse drug reactions – Causes tachycardia and hypertension.

6. Carvedilol?

Ans) It is a β1 + β2 + α1 adrenoceptor blocker. It causes vasodilatation due to α1 blockade as well as calcium channel blockade, and has antioxidant property. It has been used in hypertension and is the β blocker especially employed as a cardioprotective in congestive cardiac failure. Oral bioavailability of carvedilol is 30%. It is primarily metabolized and has a t½ of 6–8 hrs.

7. Therapeutic uses of adrenergic drugs?

Ans) Hypertension, Angina pectoris, Cardiac arrhythmias, Myocardial infarction, Congestive cardiac failure, Dissecting aortic aneurysm, Pheochromocytoma, Thyrotoxicosis, Migraine, Anxiety, Essential tremor, Glaucoma, Hypertrophic obstructive cardiomyopathy

8. Norepinephrine actions?

Ans) Bronchodilatation, causes intestinal dilatation, Reduces blood flow to the kidneys, causes rise in blood pressure

9. Dopamine?

Ans) It is a catecholamine which constitutes 80% of the catecholamine content in the brain. In the brain dopamine functions as a neuro transmitter. It is involved in several pathways in the brain including the reward pathway. In the periphery it acts to increase the urine output and sodium excretion in the kidneys, reduces insulin production etc.

Pharmacologic uses

- To treat parkinsonism
- To treat schizophrenia

- As anti-nausea agents
- To treat restless leg syndrome
- To treat attention deficit hyperactivity disorder
- To treat Tourette syndrome – A nervous system disorder involving repetitive movements or unwanted sounds.

Its precursor is levodopa which changes to dopamine after entering the blood brain barrier. Since the dopamine gets degraded before entering the BBB in the periphery itself due to peripheral decarboxylase enzyme. Levodopa is used. Levodopa is given along with peripheral decarboxylase inhibitors like benserazide and carbidopa.

Since it increases the myocardial contractility, it is preferred in cases of cardiogenic shock. It is a better choice than noradrenaline because in addition to the increase in global blood flow, it has potential advantage of increasing renal and hepatosplanchnic blood flow.

9. Amphetamine?

Ans) Amphetamine is a central nervous system stimulant used to treat ADHD, narcolepsy and obesity; examples are dextroamphetamine and methamphetamine. By exchange diffusion and reverse transport, they mediate the release of noradrenaline from the adrenergic receptors in the brain. Since it increases the alertness, increased concentration and attention span, euphoria, talkativeness, increased work capacity it is widely abused by the athletes and have included in the dope test. It causes mainly psychological dependence and lower physical dependence. The treatment of amphetamine toxicity is administration of chlorpromazine which controls the whole adrenergic effects

10. Rationale of using terazosin in benign prostatic hypertrophy?

Ans) Terazosin is an alpha blocker which relieves the symptoms of the benign prostatic hypertrophy by relaxing the muscles of the bladder and prostate.

11. Nasal decongestants?

Ans) They act by narrowing and reducing the swelling in the blood vessels and tissues in the nose. They are alpha adrenoreceptor agonists that cause vasoconstriction. E.g.; Phenyl ephedrine, Naphazoline, Oxymetazoline, Xylometazoline etc. They are used for allergic rhinitis, common cold, sinusitis etc. The over use of nasal decongestants can cause conditions such as Rhinitis medicamentosa, Atrophic rhinitis, Anosmia and local irritations. It shouldn't be used among the patients who are on the treatment with MAO inhibitors like selegilline, tranylcypromine etc. due to risk of hypertensive crisis.

12. Uses and contra indications of beta blockers?

    Ans) Uses
    To treat hypertension

- To treat angina pectoris
- To treat cardiac arrhythmias
- Heart failure
- To treat narrow angle glaucoma and open angle glaucoma
- Pheochromocytoma
- Contra indications
- Peripheral vascular diseases
- Diabetes mellitus
- Chronic obstructive pulmonary disease
- Asthma

13. Anorectic agents?

    Ans) They are also known as anorexiants or appetite suppressants, they stimulate the hypothalamic and limbic regions to promote satiety. Used to treat obesity. Drugs used are naltrexone, bupropion, lorcaserin, phentermine etc. They are used to treat obesity.

14. Drugs used in benign prostatic hypertrophy?

    Ans) Tamsulosin, Terazosin

15. Name two uterine relaxants?

Ans) Nifedipine, Indomethacin

16. Anti-cholinergic used to treat motion sickness?

    Ans) Hyoscine, Scopolamine

17. Drugs used to treat myasthenia gravis?

    Ans) Neostigmine, Pyridostigmine

CHAPTER III

Skeletal muscle relaxants

1. Classification of skeletal muscle relaxants?

   Ans) 2 types peripherally acting and centrally acting
   <u>Peripherally acting</u>

- Directly acting e.g., Dantrolene sodium and quinine
- Neuromuscular blocking

    - Depolarising e.g., Succinyl choline, Decamethonium (Not using now)
    - Non depolarising

        - Long acting e.g., Pancuronium, Doxacurium
        - Intermediate acting e.g., Vecuronium, Atracurium
        - Short acting e.g., Mivacurium

   <u>Centrally acting</u>

- Mephesin congeners e.g., Carisoprodol, Chlormezanone
- Benzodiazepines e.g., Diazepam, Lorazepam
- GABA mimetics e.g., Baclofen, Thiocolchocoside
- Centrally acting alpha-2 agonists e.g., Tizanidine

2. Atracurium?

   Ans) Atracurium is an intermediate acting nondepolarizing competitive blockers at the neuro muscular junction. Atracurium and its cis isomer cis-atracurium eliminates by undergoing some conformational changes in the plasma called as Hoffman's elimination. Since it doesn't need kidney or liver for its eliminations it is safe in children and elderly and those who have kidney or liver dysfunction.

3. Dantrolene in malignant hyperthermia?

Ans) Dantrolene is a directly acting skeletal muscle relaxant. It depresses the excitation-contraction coupling in skeletal muscle by binding to the ryanodine receptor 1, and decreases the intracellular calcium concentration by inhibiting the calcium release from the sarcoplasmic reticulum. Since the problem in the malignant hyperthermia is the dramatically increased muscle metabolism due to an increased amount of calcium which causes the muscle to contract, ATP hydrolysis, and heat production, Dantrolene is the drug of choice of malignant hyperthermia

4. Mechanism of action of pancuronium?

Ans) Pancuronium is a long acting nondepolarizing skeletal muscle relaxant which acts by being a competitively blocking acetylcholine at the neuromuscular receptors.

5. Succinyl choline apnoea?

Ans) Pseudo choline esterase is the enzyme which degrades the succinyl choline, but in some individuals instead of typical pseudo choline esterase will be having atypical pseudo choline esterase so that the time of recovery from anaesthesia by succinylcholine will be prolonged. To nullify its effects every anaesthetist should be trained to identify succinyl choline apnoea and should be able to provide ventilator mediated respiration till the patient becomes recovered from the succinyl choline apnoea. Anti-choline esterase like edrophonium produces only partial antagonism against succinyl choline apnoea.

CHAPTER IV

Autacoids

1. Drug therapy of migraine prophylaxis?

   Ans) It can be remembered using the mnemonic ABCD

   B. Anticonvulsants: e.g., Sodium valproate, Topiramate
   C. Beta-blockers: e.g., Propranolol, Atenolol, Timolol, Metoprolol
   D. Calcium channel blockers: e.g., Verapamil, Flunarizine
   E. Tricyclic antidepressants – e.g., Amitriptyline
   F.
   G. Allopurinol?

   Ans) Pharmacodynamics: Allopurinol is in vivo converted as oxypurinol and as a xanthine analogue which act as a competitive inhibitor of xanthine oxidase which prevents the further production of uric acid and there by prevents the upcoming hyperuricemia but doesn't treat the preexisting hyperuricemia. It is also used to treat tumour lysis syndrome, and preventing recurrent calcium nephrolithiasis in patients with hyperuricosuria.
   Pharmacokinetics: It is absorbed in the gastrointestinal system. After getting converted to oxypurinol in the liver with a half-life of 1 to 2 hours it is renally excreted.

3. Prostaglandins?

   Ans) USES

- To treat hyperpyrexia
- To reduce the pain sensation
- As a supplementary meditation to treat pulmonary hypertension (PGI2 - Treprostinil)
- To maintain the patency of ductus arteriosus in neonates born with congenital heart disease till surgery is done (PGE1 - Misoprostol)

- To prevent platelet aggregation
- To treat the peptic ulcer, to increase the peristaltic movements
- To treat erectile dysfunction
- To treat Postpartum hemorrhage(PGE1)
- For induction of labour (PGE2 - Dinoprostone), For cervical priming and abortion (Dinoprost - PGF2 alpha)

4. What is the rationale to use prostaglandin for acid peptic disease?

Ans) Since the Prostaglandins inhibit the gastric acid secretion, stimulates the bicarbonate secretion and increases the gastric blood volume.

5. Disease modifying antirheumatic drugs?

Ans)

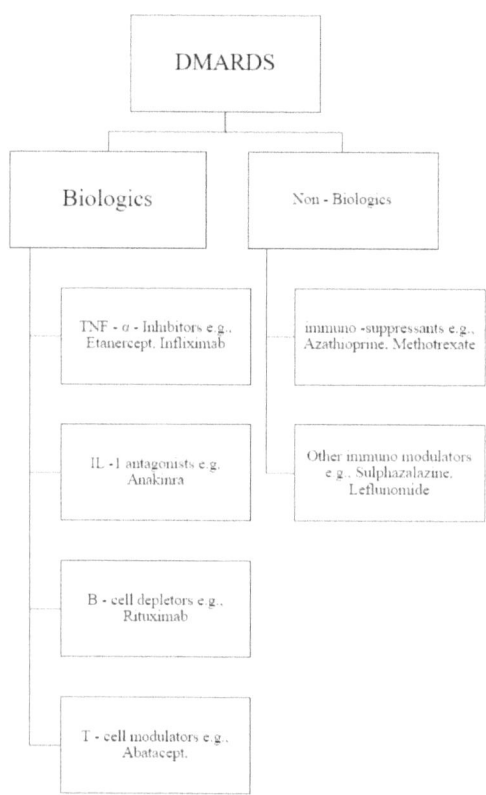

Disease modifying antirheumatoid drugs classification

6. Leflunomide?

Ans) Administered alone or with methotrexate, inhibits T cell proliferation. Its active metabolite inhibits dihydro orotate dehydrogenase, decreasing pyrimidine synthesis. Long plasma half-life of 2-3 weeks. Complete absorption even in oral dose. Loading dose is so usually given. Adverse effects - Loss of hair, Loose stools, Hepato toxic, Leukopenia. Contra indications - Lactating mother, Pregnancy, Children

7. Sumatriptan?

Ans) It is an ergot preparation coming under the group of triptans used to treat acute episodes of moderate as well as severe migraine. It is a selective 5-HT agonist.
Mechanism of action

1. $5\text{-HT}_{1D/1B}$ receptor mediated constriction of dilated cranial blood vessels especially the A-V shunts in the carotid artery which helps to divert the blood away from the brain parenchyma.
2. It inhibits the release of inflammatory peptides from the nerve endings at the perivascular space thereby reduces the inflammation there by reduces the dilatation of the arteries especially the middle meningeal artery to reduce the migraine pain by decreasing the cerebral ischemia.

Thus preferred in acute migraine. Administered orally, sub cutaneously, nasal routes. Rapid acting. Half-life 2 hours
Adverse drug reactions
It causes abnormal sensations, Discomfort in the chest with a dull ache, The skin becomes reddish and hot.
Sumatriptan is a rapidly acting triptan.

8. Second generation antihistamines?

Ans) Unlike the first-generation antihistamines the second-generation antihistamines don't crosses the blood brain barrier there by causes no sedation compared to first generation anti-histamines. Some people have reported drowsiness even with second generation antihistamines but studies comparing it with placebo have showed that it doesn't causes sedation. Additionally, they lack antiemetic effect, doesn't have any anticholinergic effects do not impair the psychomotor performance and is relatively expensive than that of first-generation antihistamines. Cetirizine is the most commonly used antihistamine which doesn't gets metabolized in our body also the incidences of cardiac arrhythmias are less with this drug. Other examples; Fexofenadine, Levocetirizine, Loratadine, Des loratadine etc.

Pharmacokinetics - They are mainly excreted via the hepatic route except for the fexofenadine, cetirizine and levocetirizine which are excreted by the renal route.

9. Non-steroidal anti-inflammatory drugs?

Ans) They mainly acts by inhibiting the cyclooxygenases which is a main intermediate in the production of prostaglandins.
They may be selective or nonselective.
<u>Nonselective cyclooxygenase inhibitors</u>
They are mainly acid derivatives including

- Salicylic acid derivatives – Acetylated - e.g., Aspirin

    Non-acetylated – e.g., Diflunisal, Salsalate.

- Propionic acid derivatives – Naproxen, Ibuprofen, Ketoprofen, Flurbiprofen
- Acetic acid derivatives – Ketorolac, Indomethacin
- Anthranilic acid derivatives - Meclofenamate, Mefenamic acid, Flufenamic acid
- Enolic acid derivatives – Piroxicam, Tenoxicam, Lornoxicam

<u>Selective cyclooxygenase inhibitors</u>
The selective cyclooxygenase inhibitors are again divided into Preferential COX-2 inhibitors and Highly selective COX-2 inhibitors

- The preferential COX-2 inhibitors include Diclofenac (Most commonly prescribed for musculoskeletal pain), Aceclofenac, Meloxicam, Nimesulide
- The highly selective COX-2 inhibitors include Celecoxib, Parecoxib, Etoricoxib

Also, there are Analgesic and anti-pyretics having weak anti-inflammatory effects like paracetamol (Most commonly prescribed over the counter drug), Nefopam

10. Naproxen?

Ans) It is a Non selective COX inhibitor NSAID, of group propionic acid derivatives. It is often given with acid blocker Nexium as it causes the release of acid from the stomach and chances for NSAID induced gastric ulcer. Given orally 500 mg b.d. Potent anti-inflammatory, inhibits migration of leukocytes. Long acting, better tolerated. Uses - To treat Rheumatoid arthritis, To treat acute gout

10. Ibuprofen?

Ans) It is the safest traditional NSAID used to treat dental surgery pains but due to its weak anti-inflammatory effects it is not used to treat inflammatory conditions like rheumatoid arthritis.

Mechanism of action – Mainly by inhibiting the both COX isoforms, in addition ibuprofen scavenges $HO^.$, $NO^.$ and $ONOO^-$ radicals and can potentiate or inhibit nitric oxide formation through its effects on Nitric oxide synthase isoforms.

11. What is the difference in the treatment of chronic gout and acute gout?

Ans) Acute gout treatment aims at immediately reduce the symptoms of inflammations so the drugs used are NSAIDs, Colchicosides etc. whereas the treatment of chronic gout aims at the cause reduction using uricosuric drugs like probenecid.

12. Acute paracetamol poisoning?

Ans) It occurs due to the increased accumulation of the metabolite NABQI which is normally gets detoxified by the conjugation of glutathione, due to the exhaustion of glutathione stores. Liver tenderness, hepatic and renal necrosis, hypoglycaemia are seen as signs. Treatment is by gastric lavage using active charcoal, and other supportive measures. The specific antidote is N-acetyl cysteine which replenishes the glutathione stores.

13. What are the adverse effects and therapeutic uses of Salicylates?

    Ans) Therapeutic uses

- To treat musculoskeletal pain
- To treat dysmenorrhoea
- To treat pain due to dysmenorrhoea
- To reduce the temperature
- To treat inflammation
- In the treatment of myocardial infarction, Heart attack, or stroke (Low dose aspirin)

Adverse effects

- Gastro intestinal symptoms like Nausea, Vomiting, Acute gastritis, it can cause gastro intestinal bleeding.
- It can be reduced by prescribing proton pump inhibitors along with NSAIDs, by taking the NSAIDs after taking food, using buffered aspirin, Using selective COX-2 inhibitors.
- Since it blocks the prostaglandin synthesis and in pregnant woman prostaglandins are essential for the uterine contractility and cervical ripening it increases the occurrences of delayed labour and postpartum haemorrhage.
- Administration of prostaglandins to mother can also cause premature closure of the ductus arteriosus again due to decrease in the prostaglandins.
- Use of salicylates in children with viral infections such as chickenpox or flu can lead to Reye's syndrome - which is a rare but serious condition which causes confusion, swelling in the brain, and liver damage.
- Due to hypersensitivity, it can cause rhinitis, bronchospasm, angioneurotic oedema.

14. What are the differences between aspirin and celecoxib?

    Ans)

Aspirin	Celecoxib
It is a nonselective COX inhibitor	It is a preferential COX-2 inhibitor
Also helps to thin the blood and prevent blood clots	Doesn't have this effect
Gastro intestinal side effects are noted	Low gastro intestinal side effects

    Differences between aspirin and celecoxib

15. Mention the mechanism of action and advantages of propionic acid derivatives?

    Ans) <u>Mechanism of Action</u>

    By inhibiting the cyclooxygenase enzymes COX1 and COX2. These enzymes catalyse the production of prostaglandins, which are responsible for pain and inflammation symptoms. By inhibiting these enzymes, propionic acid derivatives reduce the production of prostaglandins, thereby reducing pain and inflammation

    <u>Advantages</u>

    - Anti-inflammatory and Analgesic Effects
    - These drugs can reduce body temperature in fever.
    - Propionic acid derivatives are generally better tolerated than aspirin, with milder side effects and a lower incidence rate.
    - They are used in a wide range of conditions, including rheumatoid arthritis, osteoarthritis, dysmenorrhoea, and other musculoskeletal disorders.

16. Advantages of selective COX-2 inhibitors over nonselective COX inhibitors?

Ans) They cause fewer stomach and intestinal problems such as bleeding and ulcers.

17. Warfarin along with aspirin?

Ans) Warfarin is a functional vitamin k depletor so it can cause haemorrhage, aspirin also causes bleeding due to its anti-platelet effect which causes a synergic effect and there by causes haematemesis. In the cases of poisoning with warfarin the treatment is administration of vitamin k. Occasions like these can be prevented by prescribing other drugs which doesn't cause bleeding to the patient on warfarin treatment as per the consultant physician.

18. Drugs used to treat vertigo?

Ans) Cinnarizine, Betahistine (Antihistamines)

19. Treatment of dry cough and productive cough?

Ans) For productive cough - Pharyngeal demulcents like Glycerine, Lozenges syrups and Expectorants like Potassium citrate and Potassium iodide which are secretion enhancers and Mucolytics like Bromhexine, Ambroxol

For dry cough – Antitussives which are cough centre suppressants are used it is of 3 classes

Opioids e.g., Codeine, Ethylmorphine

Nonopioids – Noscapine, Dextromethorphan

Antihistaminic like Chlorpheniramine, Diphenhydramine and along with it adjuvants like Bronchodilators like Salbutamol and Terbutaline are used.

CHAPTER V

Cardiovascular system

Antihypertensives

1. Enumerate five groups of anti-hypertensive drugs with examples of each?

   Ans)

   - Angiotensin converting enzyme inhibitors: Captopril, Lisinopril, Rmipril
   - Angiotensin receptor blockers: Losartan, Telmisartan, Valsartan, Candesartan
   - Direct renin blockers: Aliskiren, Enalkiren, Remikiren
   - Calcium channel blockers: Amlodipine, Nicardipine, Felodipine
   - Diuretics: Hydrochlorthiazide (Dealt detail in renal pharmacology)

2. Explain the pharmacological basis of using diuretics to treat hypertension?

   Ans) Diuretics increase urine production by the kidneys, leading to the excretion of excess sodium and water. This reduction in blood volume decreases the pressure on arterial walls.
   Some diuretics, particularly thiazides, also cause vasodilation (relaxation of blood vessels), which further helps to lower blood pressure.

3. Mention two anti-hypertensives used in pregnancy?

   Ans) Methyl dopa, Labetalol

4. Clonidine?

Ans) Clonidine is a centrally acting antihypertensive drug.

MOA - It stimulates the Alpha - 2A receptors in vasomotor centre which reduces the sympathetic outflow from the vasomotor centres. Which causes reduction in the Cardiac output and Heart rate which inturn reduces the BP

Uses -

- To treat hypertension
- To reduce postmenopausal hot flushes
- For prophylaxis of migraine
- As preanesthetic agent

Adr - Brady cardia, Sedation, depression, dryness of mouth and eyes

5. Losartan?

Ans) Pharmacodynamics: Losartan is an angiotensin receptor blocker. It competitively blocks the binding of Angiotensin 2 to the angiotensin 1 receptor subtypes.

Pharmacokinetics - They are better tolerated than that of angiotensin converting enzymes inhibitors because of the difference that it doesn't increases the bradykinin levels which are causing the adverse drug reactions like cough so used when angiotensin enzyme inhibitors are not tolerated due to its adverse effects.

Uses - They are used in the treatment of Hypertension, Myocardial infarction, Congestive cardiac failure and diabetic nephropathy.

Adverse drug reactions - Causes hyperkalaemia in patients with renal dysfunction and those on potassium sparing diuretics, Causes hypotension, weakness, head ache, rashes, teratogenic effects so not advisable for pregnant ladies.

6. Ramipril? (Angiotensin converting enzyme inhibitors)

Ans) Ramipril is an angiotensin converting enzyme inhibitor the group of drugs which are used as first line anti-hypertensive drugs.

Pharmacodynamics: As the name suggests it blocks the conversion of angiotensin 1 to angiotensin 2 by blocking the angiotensin converting enzyme.

The functions of angiotensin 2 are

- Constriction of arterioles
- Production of aldosterone
- Stimulation of the sympathetic nervous system

When angiotensin converting enzyme inhibitors are used the above functions are not done so arterioles get dilated, aldosterone production is reduced so that the sodium and water retention of them are reduced thereby causes reduction in BP. The angiotensin converting enzymes are also involved in the degradation of bradykinin which is a potent vasodilator so the inhibition of the enzyme blocks the degradation of the bradykinin there by promotes vasodilation and reduction of BP.

Pharmacokinetics: Low first pass metabolism so that can be given orally. They get metabolized in liver.

Uses:

- To treat hypertension
- To treat coronary artery disease
- To treat certain chronic kidney diseases
- To treat heart attacks

<u>Adverse drug reactions:</u> Can be remembered by the name of another important drug in this group called CAPTOPRIL.

C – Cough
A – Angioedema
P – Pregnancy problems (Teratogenic effects)
T – Taste changes
O – Other (Rashes and fatigue)
P – Proteinuria
R – Renal insufficiency
I – Increased potassium
L – Low blood pressure.

• • •

ANTI ANGINAL DRUGS

1. Classify drugs used in the treatment of angina pectoris?

Ans)

- Nitrates

    - Short acting e.g., Glyceryl trinitrate and Isosorbide dinitrate through sublingual route
    - Long acting e.g., Isosorbide dinitrate through oral route, Isosorbide mononitrate

- Calcium channel blockers - Amlodipine, Nicardipine,
- Potassium channel openers – Nicorandil, Minoxidil
- Beta adrenergic blockers – Propranolol, Atenolol, Metoprolol
- Others e.g., Dipyridamole, Ranolazine

2. Write about nitrates and the angina treatment?

Ans) Nitroglycerin is administered by sublingual route in cute attack of Angina pectoris. Effect on coronary blood flow – By the epicardial coronary dilation, Stenosis enlargement, Enhanced collateral size and flow, improvement of endothelial dysfunction, and prevention or reversal of coronary blood flow nitrates increases the coronary blood flow.

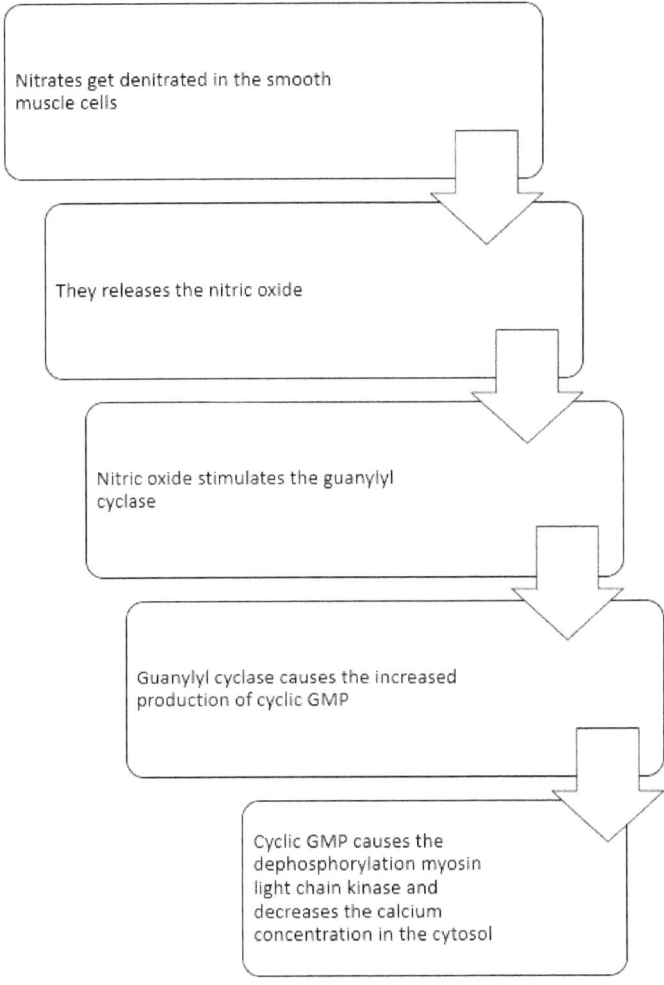

Mechanism of action of nitrates

Which causes the arteriolar and venodilatation and decreases the afterload and preload which relieves angina

<u>Adverse effects</u>

Due to the vasodilatory action of nitrates

- Headache
- Cutaneous flushing

- Hypotension
- Syncope
- Reflex tachycardia
- Methemoglobinemia

3. Beta blockers in angina?

Ans) Betablockers acts by blocking the beta-adrenergic receptors in the heart which blocks the action of hormones like adrenaline. Thereby it reduces the activity of heart causes reduced heart rate and decreased force of contraction so that the oxygen requirement of the heart (myocardium) is reduced. For example, Atenolol, Propranolol, Sotalol, Carvedilol, Bisoprolol, Labetalol, Metoprolol. Beta blockers are given as prophylactic to peoples with recent myocardial infarction and should be continued indefinitely since it reduces the mortality also it helps to increase the exercise tolerance.

Betablockers have adverse effects of bronchospasm in patients with bronchial asthma, Increases the left ventricular end-diastolic volume causes bradycardia, heart block.

The left ventricular volume rise when usage of beta blockers can be counteracted by using betablockers along with nitrates, which is the rationale for using betablockers in combination with nitrates

4. Calcium channel blockers?

Ans)

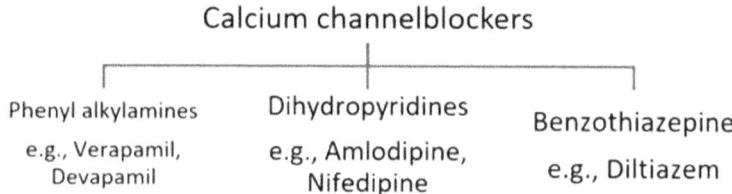

Calcium channel blockers can be used in angina since it reduces the oxygen consumption by the heart by decreasing heart rate, blood pressure and contractility.

Drug interactions – Calcium channel should not be given along with propranolol because both causes cardiac depression and when used together, they can lead to cardiac arrest.

5. Rationale of low dose aspirin in post MI?

Ans) Since in low dose aspirin acts as an anti-platelet drug so it thins the blood which prevents the formation of further blood clots.

6. Nicorandil?

Ans) Nicorandil is a potassium channel opener which can be used in the treatment of angina.
By opening the ATP dependent potassium channels, it causes the hyper polarisation at the blood vessels which will lead to the arteriolar and venodilation. It causes the release of nitric oxide which increases the cyclic GMP which aids the relaxation of vascular smooth muscles and arteriolar dilatation

7. Can propranolol be used in a patient under insulin treatment for treating hypertension? Why?

Ans) No. Because propranolol may interfere with glucose recovery after insulin-induced hypoglycaemia in diabetic patients by interfering with glucose recovery after insulin-induced hypoglycaemia in diabetic patients by blocking epinephrine's inhibition of glucose utilization. Also it masks the symptoms of hypoglycemia and causes hypoglycemic unawareness.

8. How should a hypertensive patient under insulin therapy should be treated?

Ans) In the order of best choices.
They can be treated by ACE inhibitors like Captopril, Enalapril
By calcium channel blockers like amlodipine, diuretics and beta blockers.

9. Hypertensive emergencies?

Ans) It means systolic BP greater than 180mmHg and/or diastolic BP greater than 120 mmHg

Treatment is done using Nicardipine, Sodium nitroprusside and Labetalol. Note that BP shouldn't be reduced more than 25% in first hour.

(Mnemonic hypertension is more common in elders remember the drugs as SeNiLe)

10. What is the role of propranolol in myocardial infarction?

Ans) Propranolol improves myocardial oxygenation in patients with uncomplicated acute infarction without endangering perfusion of other vital organs.

11. List the drug to be started immediately after acute myocardial infarction?

Ans)

- Aspirin if allergic Clopidogrel (Orally)
- Morphine (Intra venously), anti-emetics to address the morphine induced vomiting.
- Nitroglycerin (Intravenously),
- Low molecular weight heparins (Reviparin, Enoxaparin etc.)
- Statins (Atorvastatin, Simvastatin etc.)

12. Write the mechanism of action and two adverse effects of fibrinolytics?

Ans) Mechanism of action: It increases the speed of degradation of fibrin by aiding the conversion of fibrin-bound plasminogen to fibrin by binding to the fibrin-bound plasminogen. E.g., Streptokinase, Urokinase.

Adverse effects: Bleeding and embolization

13. Name and explain the analgesics used to relieve pain in acute myocardial infarction and its rationale for the same?

Ans) Morphine is the drug of choice due to its reliable and predictable effects, safety profile, and ease of reversibility using Naloxone. The opioid pethidine is contraindicated in myocardial infarction (MI). Since it has sympathomimetic effects that can increase heart rate and blood pressure, which may exacerbate the condition in MI patients. Morphine is the DOC even the patient have associated DM or HTN.

Dosage: 2-4 mg intravenously (IV).

Administration: Administered slowly and titrated to effect. It can be repeated every 5-15 minutes as needed, with a maximum total dose of 20 mg.

Mechanism of action of morphine - The morphine acts by binding to the mu, kappa, and delta opioid receptors. Primarily through mu receptors. After binding to these receptors it activates the GPCR coupled mechanisms. Which leads to the inhibition of the enzyme adenylate cyclase and reduces the conversion of ATP to cAMP. Morphine inhibits the opening of voltage-gated calcium channels, reducing the influx of calcium ions into the presynaptic neuron.This results in decreased release of excitatory neurotransmitters such as substance P, glutamate, and other pain-related neurotransmitters.The activation of mu receptors also leads to euphoria and sedation, contributing to its pain-relieving properties.

Morphine opens potassium channels, causing an efflux of potassium ions. This hyperpolarizes the neuron, making it less likely to fire action potentials.By reducing neurotransmitter release and decreasing neuronal excitability, morphine effectively relieves pain.

14. Drugs used in the management of acute myocardial infarction with rationale?

Ans) As a pain killer – To reduce pain because adequate pain control modulates sympathetic nervous system activation and therefore decreases myocardial oxygen demand - Morphine

As an antiemetic – As morphine can stimulate nausea and vomiting - Metoclopramide

As anti-thrombotic – To prevent thrombi associated with myocardial infarction and inhibit platelet function by blocking cyclooxygenase and subsequent platelet aggregation - Aspirin, Clopidogrel

Betablockers –Since it decreases myocardial contractility, heart rate, and elevated blood pressure, which reduce myocardial oxygen demand - Metoprolol

Anti-coagulants –Since it reduces thrombus formation- Enoxaparin, Fondaparinux

Nitrates – Because it causes vasodilation and increases the blood flow to myocardium - Isosorbide dinitrate, Glyceryl trinitrate

Calcium channel blockers – Reduce both myocardial infarct size and the incidence of ventricular arrhythmia.

...

DRUGS FOR HEART FAILURE

1. What are the first line drugs in congestive cardiac failure?

    Ans) ACE inhibitors and beta blockers

2. What is the rationale for use of each of them in congestive cardiac failure?

    Ans) ACE inhibitors relax blood vessels which lowers the blood pressure and increases the supply of blood and oxygen to the heart. The beta blockers prolong the survival rates, prevents arrhythmia, improves symptoms of heart failure and left ventricular ejection fraction.

3. Drugs used in congestive cardiac failure?

    Ans) Due to the difficulties in drawing classification in 1 table here it is plotted as 2

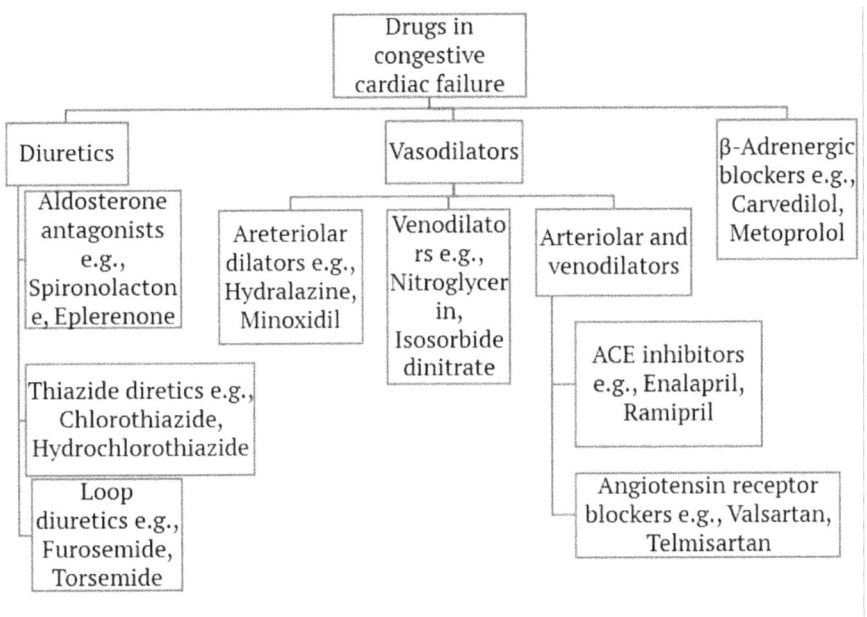

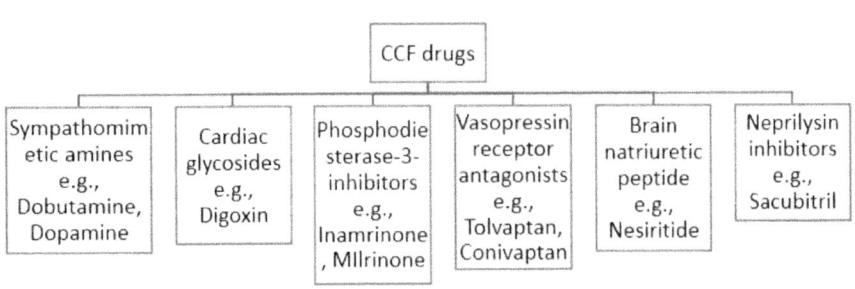

4. Role of phosphodiesterase-3-inhibitors in ccf?

Ans) It inhibits the degradation of cAMP by the enzyme phosphodiesterase-3 there by increases intracellular cAMP levels which causes a positive inotropic effect. It can also cause vasodilation by increasing cAMP in vascular smooth muscle cells, which helps reduce the workload on the heart.

5. Two uses and adverse effects if inodilators?

Ans) Uses – To treat congestive cardiac failure, to reduce the risk of intracardiac stasis.

ADR – Decreased appetite, Vomiting or diarrhoea and increased liver enzymes.

6. Mention the life style modification that you would advise to a congestive cardiac failure patient?

Ans)

- Cessation of smoking and alcoholism
- Do adequate exercise daily
- Manage stress
- Restrict salt intake

6. Add a note on treatment of digoxin over dosage?

Ans)

- The patient should be shifted to the intensive care unit
- Digoxin should be stopped, since hypokalaemia aggravates the toxicity thiazide diuretics and loop diuretics if taking should be discontinued
- Propranolol is used to treat supra ventricular arrhythmias, and lignocaine for ventricular arrhythmia
- Atropine and cardiac pacing to treat AV block and bradyarrhythmia
- Serious cases use digoxin antibodies like Digi bind

• • •

Anti-arrhythmic drugs

1. Lidocaine or Propranolol to treat arrhythmia following myocardial infarction?

    Ans) Beta blockers like propranolol are best for treating arrhythmias for reducing post myocardial infarction mortality.

2. Lignocaine in ventricular arrhythmia?

    Ans) Because it reduces the ventricular tachycardia by suppressing multiple ventricular extrasystoles.
    Dose – 1-1.5mg/Kg slow IV bolus over 2-3 minutes. May repeat doses 0.5 -0.75 mg/Kg in 5-10 minutes up to 3 mg/kg total if refractory ventricular fibrillation or pulseless ventricular tachycardia. It is a class 1B anti-arrhytmic acts by blocking the open and inactive sodium channels.

3. Drug of choice in atrial fibrillation?

    Ans) Esmolol, Verapamil

4. Drug of choice in paroxysmal supra ventricular tachycardia?

    Ans) Adenosine, Propranolol

CHAPTER VI

Respiratory system

1. Treatment of Status Asthmaticus (Refractory asthma)?

   Ans)

   - First start the treatment with 100mg Hydrocortisone hemi-succinate intravenously
   - Then nebulise the patient with salbutamol 2.5 to 5 mg and ipratropium bromide 0.5 mg with intermittent inhalations driven by oxygen
   - Give high flow humidified oxygen through inhalatory route
   - Even though we have given salbutamol inhalation it may not reach the smaller bronchi so that it is also administered intramuscularly or subcutaneously 0.4 mg
   - Intubation and mechanical ventilation are done if needed
   - If having chest infection with intensive antibiotic therapy
   - The patient may be gone to respiratory acidosis, treat the acidosis with saline and sodium bicarbonate or lactate infusion.

2. Montelukast or Salbutamol in acute bronchial asthma?

   Ans) Salbutamol, Since Montelukast cannot treat an acute asthma attack since it establishes its effect tardy.

3. Ipratropium bromide?

   Ans) It is an anticholinergic medication which opens up the medium and large airways in the lungs.
   Pharmacokinetics – Its metabolism happens in the liver
   Uses – To treat COPD (Used as inhaler)
   Adverse drug reactions – Dry mouth, Cough and inflammation of airways.

4. Drugs for bronchial asthma?

Ans)

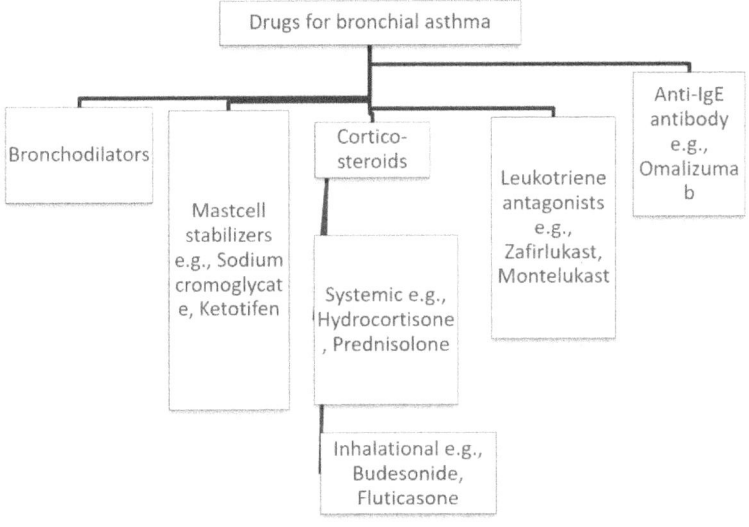

Figure 14

5. Leukotriene antagonists?

Ans) Their indication is prophylaxis and chronic treatment of asthma and exercise induced bronchoconstriction. For example, Montelukast and Zafirlukast.

Montelukast – It is a highly selective leukotriene antagonist that binds with high affinity to the cysteinyl leukotriene receptor for Leukotrienes D4 and E4. Headache is the main adverse drug reaction caused by it. Churg-Strauss syndrome is rarely seen

6. Mast cell stabilizers?

Ans) Cromoglycate - By involving a delayed chloride channel in the mast cell they stabilize the degranulation of mast cells. Its oral absorption is poor so mainly taken as inhalation. Used as a long-term prophylactic in mild to moderate bronchial asthma and for symptomatic relief of allergic rhinitis. Due to its lower water solubility its systemic absorption is poor and causes lower toxicity. But cough, throat irritation and bronchospasm are seen in some patients.

7. Bronchodilators?

   Ans)

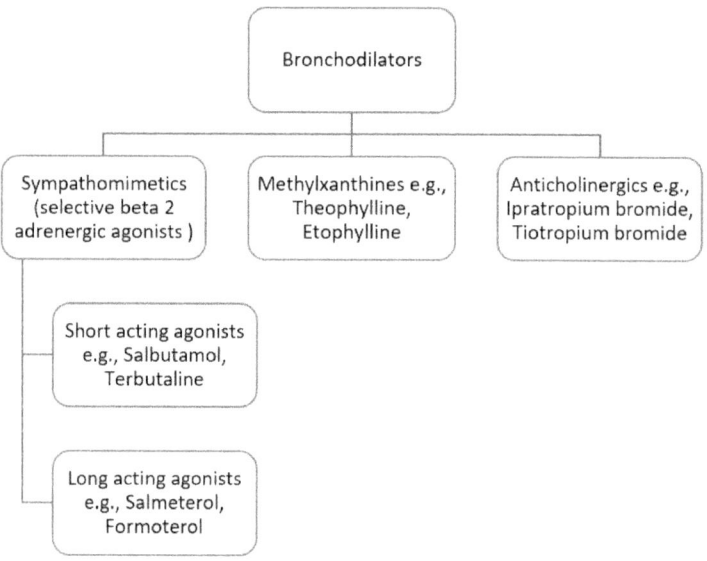

Figure 15

Mnemonic: Remember by SMA (Sympathomimetics, Methylxanthines and Anticholinergics) (Spinal muscular atrophy) Since the muscles of the bronchus are atrophied to dilate it bronchodilators are needed) Just a mnemonic not a fact.

Sympathomimetics: Mechanism of action – They stimulates the beta 2 receptors in the bronchial smooth muscles and mast cells to increase the cAMP which in turn causes bronchodilation.

Methylxanthines: They inhibits the phosphodiesterase to increase the cAMP.

Anticholinergics: In the bronchial smooth muscles, they selectively block the effects of acetylcholine to cause bronchodilation.

8. Name 2 drugs used in the treatment of acute severe bronchial asthma?

Ans) Inhalational corticosteroids and Salmeterol.

9. Theophylline?

Ans) It is a methyl xanthine which dilates the bronchi by increasing the cyclic AMP by blocking the phosphodiesterase.
ADR- It is a drug with narrow therapeutic window, Gastric pain, Rectal inflammation, Headache, Nausea, Vomiting, Nervousness are seen.

10. Name two mucolytics?

Ans) Bromhexine, Ambroxol

11. Name two antitussives?

Ans) Codeine, Noscapine. Codein is not used in case of asthmatics. Dextromethorphan is given for asthmatic patients.

12. How to instruct a patient to use metered dose inhaler?

Ans) First greet the patient and introduce yourself,
"Before taking the drug you should sit up straightly and lift the chin to open the air-ways, Shake the inhaler vigorously so as to mix its incomitances and then remove the cap, if it is used for the first time or after a time period of more than one week, spray it into the air to see whether it works, then take few breaths and breathe out gently , place the mouth piece between teeth and seal with the lips, then start breathing slowly and deeply and simultaneously press down the canister to release the drug. One press release one puff. Breathe deep to ensure that the drug reached bronchioles, remove the inhaler and hold the breath for 10 seconds and breathe out, then replace the cap on the mouth piece, Spacers are used in patients who cannot coordinate breathe and inhalation simultaneously, if the inhaler is containing corticosteroids rinse the oral cavity with water after to prevent oral candidiasis, if more than one puff is to be taken wait for 30 seconds shake the inhaler and repeat the steps, the inhaler and spacer should clean periodically."

13. Asthma mediators?

Ans) Histamine, Prostaglandins, leukotrienes, platelet activating factor, adenosine, bradykinin and sensory neuropeptides.

CHAPTER VII

Blood

1. Hypolipidemic drugs?

Ans)

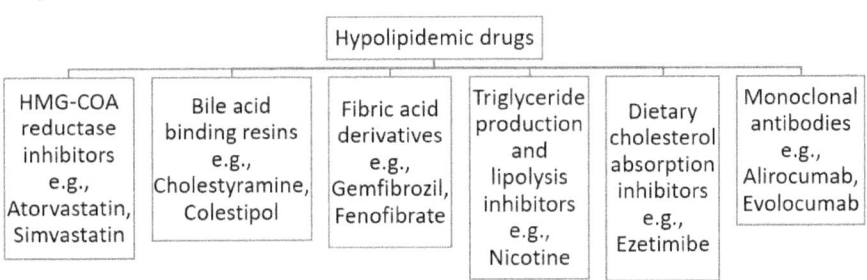

Figure 16

2. Ezetimibe mechanism of action?

Ans) Reduces the cholesterol absorption by blocking a specific cholesterol transport protein called NPC1L1 in the intestinal mucosa.

3. Human erythropoietin (Epoietin)?

Ans) It is a glycoprotein produced by kidneys which is essential factor for the viability and proliferation of erythrocytic progenitors.

4. Fibrinolytic drug?

Ans) Also known as thrombolytics.

They increase the degradation of fibrin by converting the plasminogen to plasmin. E.g., Alteplase, Tenecteplase, Streptokinase, Urokinase

Uses – Acute myocardial infarction (Tenecteplase is preferred over Alteplase in ST elevation MI), Pulmonary embolism, Deep vein thrombosis

Contra indications – Severe hypertension, Severe diabetes mellitus, Severe liver damage (As its excretion takes place mainly through the liver), Peptic ulcer, Bleeding disorders, Recent trauma or surgery.

Adverse effects – Allergic reactions, Epistaxis, Kidney failure, Low BP

5. Classification of anti-platelet drugs?

Ans) Thromboxane synthesis inhibitors e.g., Aspirin

$P2Y_{12}$ receptor blockers e.g., Clopidogrel, Prasugrel

Platelet cyclic AMP enhancers e.g., Dipyridamole

GP 2b/3a antagonists e.g., Abciximab, Eptifibatide

6. Clopidogrel?

Ans) Clopidogrel is an antiplatelet drug. Which acts by antagonising the purinergic receptor irreversibly there by blocks the ADP mediated platelet aggregation.

Uses – Transient ischaemic attack, Coronary artery disease, Acute coronary syndrome

Adverse drug reactions – Bleeding, Thrombocytopenia, Neutropenia, Diarrhoea

7. Heparin?

Ans) It is a sulphated mucopolysaccharide which is commercially obtained from the ox lung and pig intestinal mucosa. It binds to plasma anti-thrombin-3 and activates it. At low doses – It prevents the thrombus formation by inhibition of the conversion of prothrombin to thrombin.

At high doses – It prolongs the bleeding time by its antiplatelet function. It has high first pass metabolism so not effective orally. Protamine sulphate which is cationic is used in heparin over dosage because protamine binds tightly to heparin, which is higly anionic, thereby neutralizing the anticoagulant effect of Heparin.

8. Low molecular weight heparin?

Ans) They are obtained by fractionating the standard heparin. They block the coagulation cascade by inactivating factor Xa. e.g., Dalteparin, Enoxaparin

UFH (Unfractionated Heparin)	Low molecular weight heparin
aPTT monitoring required	aPTT monitoring not required
Effects are completely reversed by protamine sulfate	Effects are not completely reversed by protamine sulfate
Shorter $t_{1/2}$ and low bioavailability	Longer $t_{1/2}$ and higher bioavailability
Higher incidence of osteoporosis and thrombocytopenia	Lower incidence of osteoporosis and thrombocytopenia

Table 6

9. Two differences between heparin and warfarin?
Ans)

Heparin	Warfarin
Naturally seen	Synthetic
Active inside and outside of body system	Active only inside body system

Table 7

10. Iron therapy?

Ans) Ferrous form of iron is better absorbed than ferric form. Ascorbic acid increases the iron absorption. Excess iron is stored as ferritin. Iron is transported with the help of transferrin. Adr are Nausea and vomiting, Diarrhoea, Constipation, Acute kidney injury. Oral iron formulations includes Ferrous sulphate, Ferrous fumarate, Ferrouss gluconate. Intravenous iron formulations include Iron Dextran, Iron Sucrose, Ferric carboxymaltose. Intravenous Desferrioxamine is given in case of acute iron poisoning. The formula used for calculating the dose of parenteral iron is Total dose in milligrams equals the Body weight in Kilograms multiplied by Iron deficit in mg/Kg

11. Name two oral anticoagulants?

Ans) Dicumarol, Warfarin sodium

12. Name two direct factor Xa inhibitors?

Ans) Rivaroxaban, Apixaban

13. Name two plasma expanders?

Ans) Human albumin, Dextran

CHAPTER VIII

Renal pharmacology

1. Classify diuretics?

   Ans)

   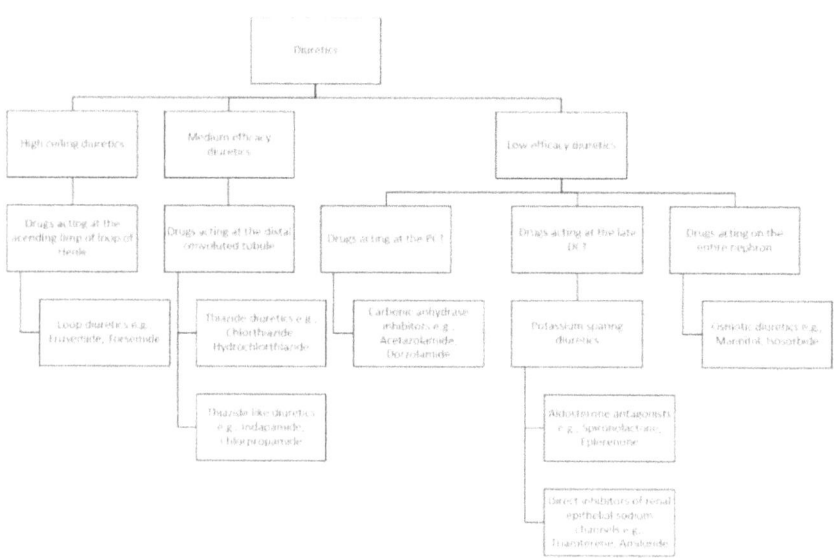

2. Frusemide uses and adverse effects?

   Ans)

Uses	Adverse effects
To treat acute pulmonary oedema	Hypokalaemia, Hyponatremia, Hypocalcaemia
To treat hypertensive emergencies	Hyperglycaemia, Hyperlipidaemia, Hyperuricaemia
To treat hypercalcaemia	Ototoxicity, Hypersensitivity

Table : Frusemide uses and adr

3. Spironolactone?

Ans) Spironolactone is a potassium sparing diuretic with acts as a competitive antagonist of the aldosterone. It acts on the late distal tubules and collecting duct. It causes potassium retention and sodium and calcium excretion.

USES	Adverse drug reactions
Hypertension – To treat hypertension due to Conn's syndrome	Hyperkalaemia
To treat congestive heart failure	Gastrointestinal side effects – Nausea, Vomiting
To treat oedema due to hyperaldosteronism in cases of Hepatic cirrhosis, Nephrotic syndrome, Congestive cardiac failure	Due to lack of action of aldosterone can cause irregular menstrual cycles and reduction of male secondary sexual characteristics and gynaecomastia

Table : Spironolactone uses and adr

4. Thiazides or Spironolactone in patients using Lisinopril?

Ans) Thiazides because since spironolactone is a potassium sparing diuretic and lisinopril is an angiotensin converting enzyme inhibitor which increases the potassium combining them may cause increase of the potassium levels to a dangerous level.

5. Furosemide?

Ans) Furosemide is a loop diuretic which acts on the thick ascending limb of loop of Henle.

Mechanism of action

The frusemide blocks the sodium potassium 2 chloride co transport to the tubular cell and thereby reducing the reabsorption of them and increases the excretion of the sodium and potassium which leads to the adverse effects hyponatremia and hypokalaemia.

It also blocks the reabsorption of calcium and magnesium to the interstitial lumen thereby increases their excretion also and causes hypocalcaemia and hypomagnesemia, the disruptions of electrolytes lead to ototoxicity.

Mechanism of action –

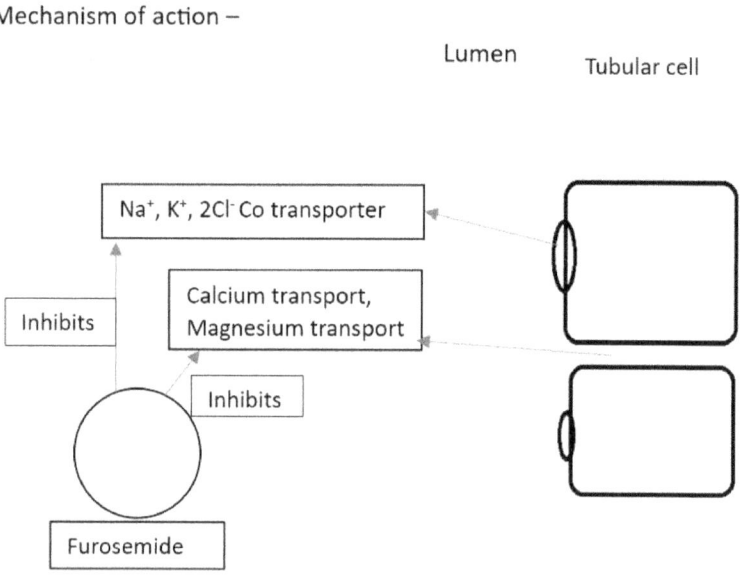

Figure : Mechanism of action of Loopdiuretics

Frusemide uses and adr

Uses	Adverse effects
To treat acute pulmonary oedema	Hypokalaemia, Hyponatremia, Hypocalcaemia
To treat hypertensive emergencies	Hyperglycaemia, Hyperlipidaemia, Hyperuricaemia
To treat hypercalcaemia	Ototoxicity, Hypersensitivity

Table : Frusemide uses and adr

Frusemide in pulmonary edema

```
┌─────────────────────────────┐
│ Increases the prostaglandin │
│    synthesis and release    │
└─────────────────────────────┘
              ↓
┌─────────────────────────────┐
│   Prostaglandin causes      │
│        vasodilation         │
└─────────────────────────────┘
              ↓
┌─────────────────────────────┐
│ The blood from the pulmonary│
│ vessels get transferred to  │
│    the peripheral vessels   │
└─────────────────────────────┘
              ↓
┌─────────────────────────────┐
│  Pulmonary edema is relieved│
└─────────────────────────────┘
```

CHAPTER IX

Central nervous system

LOCAL ANAESTHETICS

1. Rationale of using adrenaline with local anaesthetics?

   Ans) Adrenaline causes vasoconstriction thereby decreases the distribution of local anaesthetics to distant places through blood increases its duration of action, reduces the dose of anaesthetic needed thereby reduces the systemic toxicity. It also helps to create a blood free field for the action of local anaesthetics.

2. Mechanism of action of lignocaine?

   Ans)

```
┌─────────────────────────────────────┐
│ Lignocaine being a weak base exists │
│ as partly ionised and unionised form│
└─────────────────────────────────────┘
                  ↓
┌─────────────────────────────────────┐
│ The partly unionised form enters the│
│            nerve cells              │
└─────────────────────────────────────┘
                  ↓
┌─────────────────────────────────────┐
│ Inside the nerve cells it again gets│
│      converted in to ionised form   │
└─────────────────────────────────────┘
                  ↓
┌─────────────────────────────────────┐
│ It enters the sodium channel in the │
│       open state of the channel     │
└─────────────────────────────────────┘
                  ↓
┌─────────────────────────────────────┐
│   It binds to the sodium channel    │
│   from inside in the closed state   │
└─────────────────────────────────────┘
                  ↓
┌─────────────────────────────────────┐
│    Prolongs the inactivated state   │
└─────────────────────────────────────┘
                  ↓
┌─────────────────────────────────────┐
│    Decreases the action potential   │
└─────────────────────────────────────┘
                  ↓
┌─────────────────────────────────────┐
│       Causes local anaesthesia      │
└─────────────────────────────────────┘
```

Flowchart : Mechanism of action of Lignocaine

• • •

General anesthetics

1. Propofol?

Ans) It is an anaesthesia inducing drug which is administered parenterally.

Mechanism of action

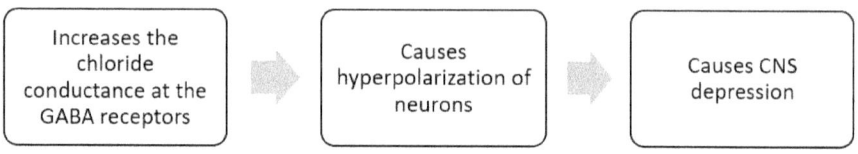

Flowchart : Propofol mechanism of action

Uses and advantages

- It is the general anaesthetic commonly used for outpatient procedures
- It has antiemetic effect so reduces the post operative vomiting
- Rapid induction and recovery from anaesthesia
- Aids in both induction and maintenance of anaesthesia
- For the treatment of status asthmaticus if not controlled by other drugs.

Disadvantages

- Causes fall in BP and respiratory depression

2. Ketamine?

Ans) It is a slower acting general anaesthetic which acts by blocking the NMDA type of excitatory amino acid receptors in the brain.

It produces a special type of anaesthesia called dissociative anaesthesia in which the person feels dissociated from there body, profound analgesia, immobility and amnesia are noted with only light sleep, respiration is not depressed. Non purposive limb movements (Used in patients with hypothermia). Increased heart rate, cardiac output and elevated blood pressure can occur. Well tolerated by children

3. Pre anaesthetic medication?

Ans) Purpose – To make anaesthesia safer and more comfortable to the patient.

Drugs used

- To reduce vagal brady cardia, hypotension and to secretions (Salivary secretions can cause aspiration and may lead to aspiration pneumonia, Respiratory secretions can cause sudden laryngospasm) e.g., Glycopyrrolate
- Anxiolytics – e.g., Midazolam, Diazepam, Lorazepam
- To relieve pre anaesthetic and post anaesthetic pain opioid analgesics can be used
- To speed up the emptying of the gastric contents in case of emergency surgeries and for antiemetic action Ondansetron, Metoclopramide can be used
- To prevent stress induced gastric ulcers proton pump inhibitors like Pantoprazole or H2-blockers like ranitidine or cimetidine can be used

4. Halothane?

Ans) Halothane is an inhalational general anaesthetic which is a volatile liquid. It is highly potent and causes faster induction as well as recovery of anaesthesia and is also doesn't causes irritation or inflammation to the airways, but its analgesic as well as muscular relaxation are poor and can cause hypotension, arrhythmias and is expensive.

5. Sevoflurane?

Ans) Similar to halothane

6. Inhaled anesthetics vs intravenous anesthetics?

Ans)

Intravenous anaesthetics	Inhaled anaesthetics
It is extensively used in outpatients	Less use in outpatients
Onset is faster	Slow onset
Specialised equipments are not necessary	Specialised equipments are necessary
Examples - Thiopentone sodium, Propofol	Examples – Desflurane, Sevoflurane

Difference between inhaled and intravenous anesthetics

• • •

Ethyl and methyl alcohols

1. Disulfiram or Fomepizole in methyl alcohol poisoning?

Ans) Fomepizole, even though both blocks the aldehyde dehydrogenase enzyme fomepizole is having shorter half-life than that of disulfiram. So that patient should abstain from alcohol for a long time. So, the patient compliance and adherence are better with the use of fomepizole

2. Rationale for the use of ethanol in the treatment of methanol poisoning?

Ans) Since the ethanol competitively blocks the conversion of methanol to toxic formaldehyde by competitively blocking the enzyme alcohol dehydrogenase, preferred only when fomepizole is not available due to its erratic absorption

3. Mechanism of action of disulfiram?

Ans)

> Binds to aldehyde dehydrogenase to block the degradation of alcohol

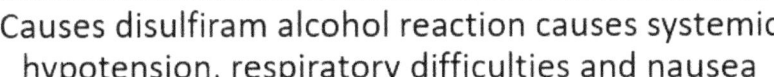

> Causes disulfiram alcohol reaction causes systemic hypotension, respiratory difficulties and nausea

· · ·

SEDATIVES AND HYPNOTICS

1. Diazepam?

   Ans) Diazepam is a benzodiazepine
   Uses

- For the treatment of anxiety disorders
- For treating preoperative anxiety
- For treating certain refractory epilepsy patients
- As an adjunct therapy in severe recurrent convulsive seizures
- As an adjunct therapy in status epilepticus
- As an adjunct therapy in alcohol detoxification

   Mechanism of action
   Facilitates the activity of GABA by increasing the frequency of opening of the chloride channels unlike barbiturates which prolongs the duration of opening of the chloride channels which leads to the hyperpolarisation of the neuronal membranes and reduced neuronal excitability.
   Adverse drug reactions

- Respiratory depression, Suicidality, Dependency, Sedation, Fatigue, Confusion

Flumazenil is a specific antidote of diazepam which acts by competitively inhibits the benzodiazepines.

2. Drugs used for treating insomnia?

Ans) Benzodiazepines, Benzodiazepine receptor agonists, Melatonin receptor agonists, Anti-depressants

• • •

Anti - Epilepticus

1. Enumerate four groups of antiepileptic drugs with examples?

Ans) (Mnemonic – HI are you BC (busy) to get Succeed in life and buy a BENZ car or else a cycle of GABA company)
   H – Hydantoins – Phenytoin, Fosphenytoin
   I – Iminostilbenes- Carbamazepine, Oxcarbazepine
   B – Barbiturates – Phenobarbitone, Amobarbital
   Deoxybarbiturate e.g., Primidone
   C – Carbolic acid derivatives – Sodium valproate, Divalproex
   S – Succinimide – Ethosuximide, Methsuximide
   BENZ – Benzodiazepines – Diazepam, Lorazepam
   Cyclic GABA analogues e.g., Gabapentin, Pregabalin
   Phenyltriazine e.g., Lamotrigene

2. Enumerate the newer drugs used in the treatment of epilepsy?

Ans)

- Topiramate
- Tiagabine
- Vigabatrin
- Zonisamide

5. Write the mechanism of action of any two newer anti-epileptic agents?

Ans) <u>Topiramate</u>

- Potentiates GABA by a post synaptic effect
- Antagonism of certain glutamate receptors
- Prolongation of sodium channel inactivation
- Suppression of repetitive neuronal firing
- Prolongation of neuronal Na+ channel reactivation
- Neuronal hyperpolarisation by k+ channels

<u>Zonisamide</u>

- Prolongation of Na+ channel inactivation resulting in suppression of repetitive neuronal firing
- Suppresses the T – type Ca^{2+} currents in certain neurones

3. Lamotrigine?

Ans) It can be used as a monotherapy or as an additional drug to treat general tonic clonic seizure, Absence seizure, Myoclonic seizure and partial seizure.

MOA - Lamotrigine delays the recovery of sodium channels from inactivation.

Adverse drug reactions include Sedation, Skin rashes, Headache and nausea, vomiting.

4. Valproic acid (Sodium valproate)?

Ans) It is a broad-spectrum anti-epileptic drug in the group carboxylic acid derivative. It is broad spectrum because it acts by 3 mechanisms

- <u>Increases the GABA activity in the brain</u>

By inhibiting the GABA-transaminase enzyme, it decreases the degradation of GABA

By stimulating the glutamic acid decarboxylase enzyme, it increases the synthesis of GABA

- In the thalamic neurons it blocks the T-type calcium current

- It delays the recovery of sodium channels from inactivation

Pharmacokinetics – It have low first pass metabolism so that completely absorbed from GIT. Excretion mainly takes place in the liver.

Uses – To treat Seizures, Bipolar disorder, Mania, and for migraine prophylaxis.

Adverse drug reactions – Vomiting, Anorexia, Acute Liver failure, Acute Pancreatitis, Skin Rashes, Oro facial abnormalities due to its Teratogenicity, Elevation of liver enzymes.

5. Carbamazepine?

Ans) Carbamazepine is an anti-epileptic of the Iminostilbenes group and it acts by slowing the rate of recovery of sodium channels. It a drug which shows autoinduction which means one of its metabolites induces its excretion. It is the drug of choice for general tonic clonic seizure and absence seizure, Acute manias, bipolar disorder and Trigeminal neuralgias.

Drug interactions – Phenytoin increases the metabolism of carbamazepine and can cause the carbamazepine to sub therapeutical levels.

Valproic acid decreases the metabolism of carbamazepine and can cause its toxicity.

Contra indications – Known hypersensitivity reactions to carbamazepine, AV block, bone marrow depression, history of hepatic porphyria.

It can cause adverse effects of Sedation, Diplopia, Ataxia, Blurred vision, Drowsiness, Vertigo, Nausea, Vomiting, Confusion.

6. Discuss the line of management of Status Epilepticus?

Ans) Even if only the management is asked it is better to write what is status epilepticus.

Seizure activity occurs for more than 30 minutes or 2 or more seizures occurs without recovery of convulsions.

- Maintain airway of the patient, correct fluid and electrolyte balance
- Administer 20 to 50 ml of 50% dextrose intravenously if the hypoglycaemia is the precipitating cause

- Lorazepam 4 mg administered intravenously (Child dosage 0.1 mg/Kg) at the rate of 2 mg/minute which is repeated after 10 minutes if required
- Diazepam 10 mg is administered intravenously which is repeated after 10 minutes if required
- Fosphenytoin 100-150mg per minute intravenously or if and only if it is not available phenytoin sodium is given at a rate of 25 to 50 mg per minute since phenytoin sodium causes marked local vascular complications
- For refractory cases which doesn't responds even after 40 minutes of doing the above-mentioned things

7. Two drugs useful in absence seizures?

   Ans) Sodium valproate and Ethosuximide
   (Mnemonic – (Malayalam) Val entho manushyanu absent aanu)

8. Drugs useful in generalised tonic clonic seizures?

   Ans) Sodium valproate and Lamotrigine (Mnemonic- Generally we all do Sleep)

9. What is the mechanism of action of phenytoin?

   Ans) Phenytoin decreases the neuronal excitability by delaying the recovery of inactivated sodium channels and inhibits high-frequency firing thereby stabilizes the neuronal membrane

• • •

Anti-parkinsonism drugs

1. Levodopa?

   Ans) Levodopa is a dopamine precursor which is used to increase the dopamine concentration in the brain in the treatment of Idiopathic parkinsonism. The reason for using precursor instead of dopamine itself is to cross the blood brain barrier and reach the basal ganglia since dopamine as such cannot cross the blood brain barrier. But there is peripheral decarboxylase enzyme which converts levodopa to dopamine even before crossing the blood brain barrier to counteract this levodopa is taken along with peripheral decarboxylase inhibitors like carbidopa or benserazide in the ratio 4:1, which also decreases the cardiovascular side effects like Hypotension, Cardiac arrhythmias, Tachycardia and increases the bioavailability of the dopamine in the basal ganglia. Also, if we are using sustained release preparation of levodopa-carbidopa the on off phenomenon of levodopa which is causing due to the reduction of the plasma concentration of the levodopa is reduced.The combination also reduces the involuntary movements and postural hypotension.

The other adverse effects caused by it are gastrointestinal side-effects like nausea, vomiting etc. alteration of taste sense, abnormal involuntary movements, euphoria, confusion, delusion, depression, anxiety are also seen.

2. Enumerate four groups of drugs used in treatment of Parkinsons disease?

Ans)

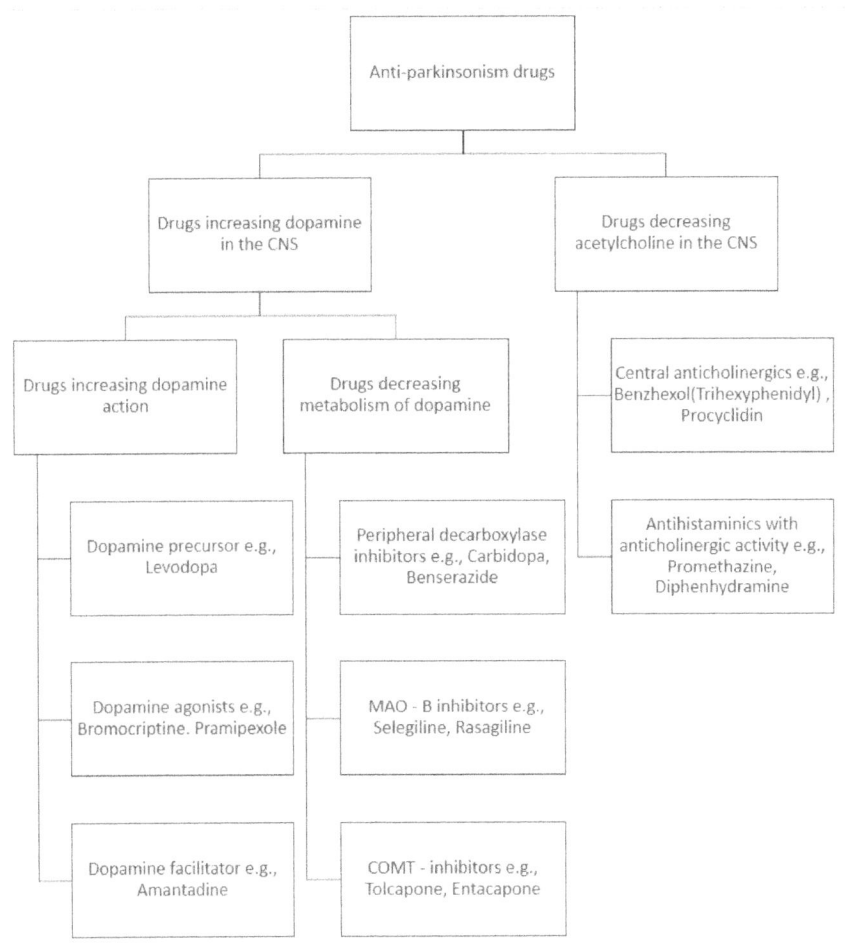

Anti-parkinsonism drugs classification

3. 2 uses and Adverse drug reactionsof Bromocriptine?

Ans)Bromocriptine is a dopamine agonist used to treat parkinsonism. It is also used to treat pituitary tumours.

Uses

- To treat Parkinson's disease
- To treat Hyperprolactinemia

<u>Adverse drug reactions</u>

- Light headedness, Compulsive behaviour

4. COMT inhibitors?

Ans) They are catechol-o-methyl transferase inhibitors which increases the availability of dopamine by blocking its metabolism to 3-o-methyl dopa by the above-mentioned enzyme. Examples are entacapone and tolcapone, Entacapone only blocks the enzyme in the peripherally whereas the tolcapone have both central and peripheral actions (Remember as tolcapone, talks to others an extrovert so both peripheral and central action and Entacapone only one place peripherally).It thereby increases the bioavailability of levodopa and half-life are prolonged with this.

Adverse effects – Diarrhoea, Nausea, Dyskinesia, Hypotension and Hallucinations.

5. What is the cause of development of rigidity, tremor, hypokinesia and festinant gait in a patient on treatment with haloperidol? And how will you treat it?

Ans) It is due to the development of extrapyramidal side effects of haloperidol; it can be treated using centrally acting anticholinergics like Benztropine and Benzhexol (Now named as Trihexyphenidyl)

• • •

DRUGS USED IN MENTAL ILLNESS

ANTI-PSYCHOTICS AND ANTI-MANIAC DRUGS

1. Atypical antipsychotic agents?

Ans) Atypical antipsychotics are drugs which blocks the 5-HT_2 receptor instead of the dopamine (D_2 receptor) as in case of typical antipsychotics. But they also have weak D_2 blocking effect. Examples are Risperidone,

Olanzapine, Clozapine etc. They have less extra pyramidal side effects. Clozapine is a reserve drug due to its dangerous side effect of agranulocytosis, used to treat resistant cases of schizophrenia. Atypical antipsychotics are mainly used in patients with high extrapyramidal side-effects due to the use of typical antipsychotics. It can cause adverse drug reactions like weight gain and cardiometabolic disturbances

2. 2 uses and 2 adverse effects of chlorpromazine?

   Ans)

Uses	Adverse effects
To treat mania	Parkinsonism
To treat intractable hiccough	Neuroleptic malignant syndrome

3. Compare and contrast Chlorpromazine and Risperidone?

   Ans)Chlorpromazine - First generatin (Typical anti-psychotic) where as Risperidone is of second generation.
   Chlorpromazine used to treat Schizophrenia, bipolar disorder, nausea, vomiting, hiccups, tetanus and acute intermittent porphyria where as Risperidone to treat Schizophrenia, bipolar disorder, autism, irritability associated with autism.
   Chlorpromazine blocks dopamine D2 receptors, blocks serotonin receptors, blocks alpha-adrenergic receptors whereas Risperidone Blocks dopamine D2 receptors, serotonin 5-HT2A receptors, alpha-adrenergic receptors
   Side-effects of Chlorpromazine are Extrapyramidal symptoms, tardive dyskinesia, sedation, orthostatic hypotension, anticholinergic effects whereas of Risperidone are Weight gain, metabolic syndrome, extrapyramidal symptoms (less common), hyperprolactinemia, sedation
   Chlorpromazine is administered Oral, intramuscular, intravenous routes whereas Risperidone Oral, oral solution, oral disintegrating tablet, intramuscular, extended-release injectable routes

4. Trihexyphenidyl and haloperidol in schizophrenia?

Ans) The combination helps to reduce side effects.

5. Lithium uses and adverse drug reactions?

   Ans) <u>Uses</u>

- To treat bipolar disorder
- To treat resistant bipolar disorder
- To treat attention deficit hyperactivity disorder
- To treat mania and hypomania

   <u>Adverse effects</u>

- Increased frequency of urine and thirst
- Slow heart beat
- Fainting
- Weight gain

Excessive intake of sodium reduces the toxicity of lithium. Its dosage may need to be reduced in patients taking diuretics since the diuretics can effect the lithium clearance. Also it has low therapeutic range so requires therapeutic drug monitoring.

6. Extra pyramidal symptoms of antipsychotics?

Ans) It includes akathisia (Feeling of restlessness with a constant desire to move), acute dystonia (Involuntary muscle contractions), Tardive dyskinesia (Involuntary repetitive movements), Centrally acting anticholinergics are used to treat.

• • •

Anti-depressants and anti-anxiety drugs

1. Amitriptyline?

Ans) Amitriptyline is a tricyclic anti-depressant used to treat low mood and depression.

2. SSRIs and their advantages?

Ans) SSRI means selective serotonin reuptake inhibitors for example fluoxetine and fluvoxamine. They inhibit the reuptake of serotonin into the neuron thereby increases the availability of serotonin in the serotonin receptors of the CNS thereby increases its activity. Administration of them with pethidine or tramadol can cause serotonin syndrome characterised by neuromuscular excitation and altered mental state. It causes no weight gain, hypotension or sedation, convulsions as other antipsychotics. But it can cause impotency, insomnia, nausea, vomiting, diarrhoea.

3. Diazepam or Alprazolam in a depressed person with anxiety?

Ans) Diazepam as it is more effective in controlling anxiety

• • •

Opioid analgesics and antagonists

1. Enumerate opioid receptors?

Ans)

- mu receptor
- kappa receptor
- delta receptor
- nociception receptor
- zeta recepor

2. Morphine?

Ans) It belongs to class opioid analgesics. It acts on the opioid receptors to induce analgesia and alter the perception and emotional response to pain. It has low oral bioavailability and metabolism happens mainly in the liver

(Other details are present in the upcoming questions)

3. Naloxone or Nalbuphine in morphine poisoning?

Ans) In the context of morphine poisoning, where respiratory depression is a major concern, naloxone is preferred because it can effectively reverse opioid-induced respiratory depression. Nalbuphine, on the other hand, may not be as effective in reversing severe respiratory depression caused by morphine overdose. The naloxone can be administered through intravenous, intramuscular, intranasal or intraosseous route. The Nalbuphine can be administered through intravenous, intramuscular or subcutaneous routes.

4. Rationale of using methadone in morphine dependent therapy?

Ans) Prevents the Abstinence Syndrome Reduces the Narcotic Cravings Blocks the Euphoric Effects

5. Use of morphine in left ventricular failure?

Ans) Morphine is used in left ventricular failure because it reduces the pulmonary congestion, causes vasodilation thereby reduces the preload of heart, and relieves the dyspnoea and anxiety.

6. Two uses and adverse effects of morphine?

Ans)

Uses	Adverse effects
To treat myocardial pain	Respiratory depression
To treat kidney stone pain	Constipation

Table : Morphine uses and adr

It is also used to treat pre-operative and post-operative pain.

7. Why morphine is contra indicated in patients with head injury? where all it is contraindicated?

Ans) Because morphine can increase the intracranial pressure, decrease the mean arterial blood pressure and cerebral perfusion pressure, causes respiratory depression which can exacerbate hypoxia and can worsen the brain injury. It is also containdicated in cases of heart falure, secondar to chronic lung disease.

8. Tramadol?

Ans) It is an opioid pain medication and a serotonin–norepinephrine reuptake inhibitor (SNRI) used to treat moderately severe pain. It is a synthetic opioid and acts in the brain and spine (central nervous system) to reduce the amount of pain that feels.

Common side effects include constipation, itchiness, and nausea. Serious side effects may include hallucinations, seizures, increased risk of serotonin syndrome, decreased alertness, and drug addiction. It is not recommended in those who are at risk of suicide or in those who are pregnant.

9. Modafinil in night shift workers?

Ans) Modafinil is a CNS stimulant. It reduces the sleepiness, and improves the performance at the same time does not affects the daytime sleep.

CHAPTER X

Chemotherapy

Anti-microbials general consideration

1. Anti-biotic resistance

Ans) Anti-biotic resistance happens when microbes develop the ability to defeat the drugs designed to kill them. For example, MRSA – methicillin resistant staphylococcus aureus is formed when the staphylococcus aureus got the ability to resist the action of benzyl penicillin. To prevent this proper antibiotic stewardship "the effort to measure and improve how antibiotics are prescribed by the physicians and used by the patients" should be implemented.

2. Super infection?

Ans) It is the occurrence of a new infection due to antimicrobial therapy to another infection. Here the causative organism should be different from the primary organism. It is happening due to the anti-microbial anti-biotics especially the broad-spectrum antibiotics alters the normal flora. Normally normal flora inhibits the pathogenic microorganisms by the production of bacteriocins and competing for the essential nutrients but due to the alterations the normal flora couldn't do it and the pathogenic microorganisms flourishes.

3. What is post antibiotic effect and mention one example?

Ans) It is the period of time after the complete removal of an antibiotic during which there is no growth of the target organism is noted. For example, prolonged post antibiotic effects have been reported after aminoglycoside or fluoroquinolone exposure of Gram-negative L. bacilli, whereas most beta-lactam antibiotics exhibit shorter post antibiotic effect.

4. Antibiotics of choice in pregnancy?

   Ans) Penicillin, Cephalosporin, Clindamycin

5. Name two anti-scabies agents?

   Ans) Permethrin, Ivermectin

• • •

Quinolones

1. Chloroquine?

   Ans) Chloroquine is chemically a 4-aminoquinoline
   It acts as

- A suppressive prophylactic and in clinical cure (erythrocytic schizonticide)
- Gametocidal for plasmodium vivax

Pharmacokinetics

- It is synthetically available as chloroquine phosphate
- It gets rapidly and completely absorbed from the gastro intestinal tract
- It is metabolised in liver
- Peak concentration is achieved in 2-3 hours after oral dose
- High tissue distribution especially in liver, spleen, lung and kidney
- Half-life is 3-4 days but terminal half-life is 1-2 months.

Mechanism of action

```
┌─────────────────────────────────────────┐
│ Chloroquine being a basic drug          │
│ accumulates in the acidic bacterial     │
│ food vaculie                            │
└─────────────────────────────────────────┘
                    ▼
┌─────────────────────────────────────────┐
│ It prevents the accumulation of heme to │
│ hemozoin so that heme accumulates which │
│ is toxic to the parasite                │
└─────────────────────────────────────────┘
                    ▼
┌─────────────────────────────────────────┐
│ Drug complex with heme disrupts the cell│
│ membrane function, intercalating with   │
│ the parasite DNA and inhibiting the DNA │
│ synthesis                               │
└─────────────────────────────────────────┘
```

Flowchart : Chloroquine mechanism of action

Uses

- To treat acute attack and as a chemoprophylactic agent of malaria caused by plasmodium vivax, plasmodium ovale, plasmodium malaria and chloroquine sensitive plasmodium vivax.
- To treat giardiasis
- To treat amoebic liver abscess – Since the concentration of the chloroquine take place in the liver.
- To treat lepra reaction due to its anti-inflammatory effect.
- To treat rheumatoid arthritis since it stabilizes the lysosomal membrane by scavenging it
- To treat infectious mononucleosis
- To treat autoimmune disorders like systemic lupus erythematosus.

Contraindications

- Myopathy
- Visual abnormalities
- Hematologic disorders
- Porphyria
- Epilepsy
- Nausea, Vomiting

<u>Adverse drug reactions</u>

- Skin rashes, Itching
- Head ache, Visual disturbances
- Hypotension, Cardiac arrhythmias, Cardiac arrest
- Neuropathy, Psychiatric disturbances, Confusion (With parenteral administration)
- Rheumatoid arthritis
- Irreversible retinopathy (Bulls eye maculopathy) and ototoxicity.

2. Fluoroquinolones?

   Ans) Classification
   <u>According to Antimicrobial spectrum</u>

First generation	Second generation	Third generation	Fourth generation
Gram-negative but pseudomonas species	Gram-negative, some gram positive and mycobacteria	Have increased activity against gram positive pathogens and mycobacteria.	Have increased activity against gram positive pathogens and mycobacteria
e.g., Nalidixic acid, Oxolinic acid	e.g., Ciprofloxacin, Levofloxacin	e.g., Galtifloxacin, Sparfloxacin (Respiratory effects	e.g., Moxifloxacin (Used in eye), Gemifloxacin

Table : Classification of fluoroquinolones

3. Ciprofloxacin?

   It is a prototype of the second-generation fluoroquinolones.
   <u>Antibiotic spectrum</u>: Effective mainly against gram negative bacteria (Against Enterobacteriaceae, Neisseria gonorrhoea, Neisseria meningitidis etc.) and some gram-positive bacteria.

Mechanism of action: They are bactericidal which acts by inhibiting the DNA gyrase and topoisomerase 4 which are required for DNA replication and transcription.

Teratogenic so not used in pregnant ladies.

Pharmacokinetics

- Route of administration - Can be administered orally, intravenously.
- Absorption – Absorbed well from the gastro intestinal system.
- Distribution – Distributed widely in the body.
- Excretion – Mainly through urine.

Uses

- Typhoid
- Urinary tract infection
- Diarrhoea
- Chancroid
- In the regimen to treat drug resistant tuberculosis
- Eye infections
- Anthrax

Adverse drug reactions

- Gastro intestinal side effects like Nausea, Vomiting and abdominal discomfort
- Hyper sensitivity reactions like Itching, Skin rashes, Urticaria

Contra indications of fluoroquinolones

- Previous allergic reactions to the drug
- Use of drugs which prolong the QT interval or significant bradycardia
- Childrens and elderly patients
- Uncorrected hypokalaemia

4. Galtifloxacin?

Ans) Galtifloxacin is a fourth-generation fluoroquinolone used to treat infections of eye such as bacterial conjunctivitis. It causes significantly less disruption of corneal wound integrity. (Write about fluoroquinolones)

• • •

BETALACTAM ANTIBIOTICS

1. Classify beta lactam antibiotics?

   Ans)

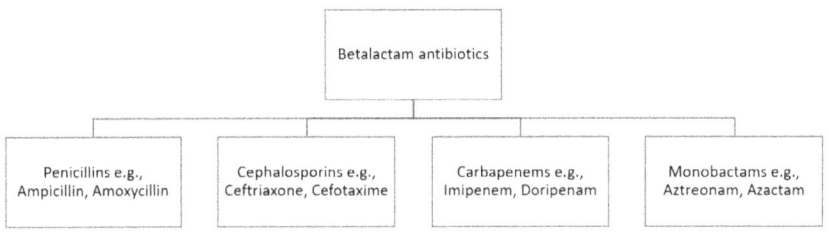

   Classification of betalactam antibiotics

2. Describe the mechanism of action of penicillin?

   Ans) Penicillin act by inhibiting the cell wall synthesis by competitively inhibiting the transpeptidase enzyme from the fourth amino acid alanine in the microbial cell wall synthesis

3. Benzyl penicillin?

   Ans) It is a preparation of naturally occurring penicillin G.
   Pharmacokinetics – Poor oral bioavailability as it gets destroyed by gastric acid (Semi-synthetic Acid resistant penicillin tackles the problem). It is having high volume of distribution due to its high tissue binding capacity. Excretion happens through kidneys, so that in infants and neonates whom the renal system is not well developed the excretion is low. Since it is excreted renally through active tubular secretion to extend its duration of action it is given along with uricosuric drugs like probenecid so that

it instead of penicillin uric acid will be excreted through active tubular reabsorption.

Spectrum of action – Spirochetes, Clostridium spp., N. meningitidis, Corynebacterium diphtheriae

Uses – To treat syphilis, diphtheria, gonococcal infections, gas gangrene

Adverse drug reactions – Allergic reactions, urticaria, dermatitis, bronchospasm

4. Classification of penicillin?

Ans)

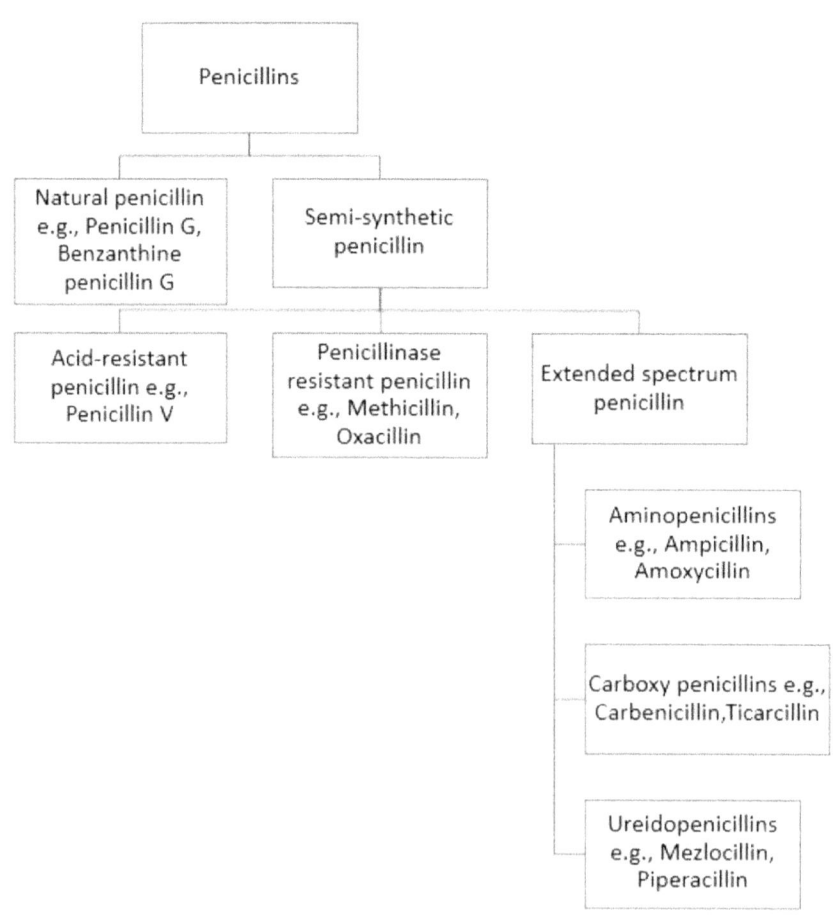

Classification of penicillin

5. Third generation or Fourth generation cephalosporins in MRSA infection?

   Ans) 4th generation cephalosporins

6. Classify cephalosporins?

   Ans)

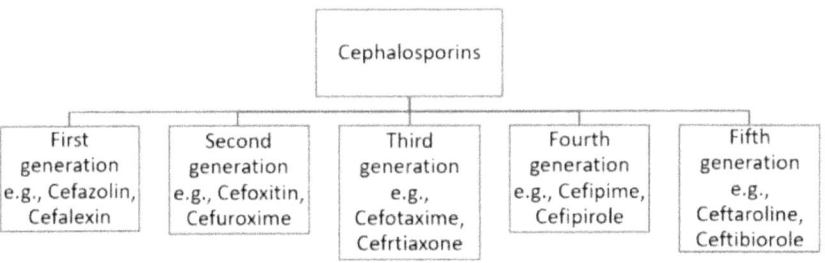

7. Second generation cephalosporins and its uses?

   Ans) These antibiotics are bactericidal.

   Mechanism of action - Similar to penicillin by binding and blocking the activity of enzymes responsible for making peptidoglycan, an important component of the bacterial cell wall.

   Second-generation cephalosporins are effective against a wide range of bacteria, including gram-negative aerobes such as Neisseria gonorrhoeae (non-penicillinase producing strains), Haemophilus influenzae, Klebsiella species, and Escherichia coli; gram-positive aerobes such as Streptococcus pneumoniae, Staphylococcus aureus, S. epidermidis and S. pyogenes; and several types of anaerobes. But most strains of Pseudomonas aeruginosa and Acinetobacter species, are resistant to second-generation cephalosporins.

   USES

- Urinary tract infections
- Lower respiratory tract infections
- Gynaecological infections
- Skin and skin structure infections
- Bone and joint infections

Second-generation cephalosporins are generally safe, with low toxicity and good efficacy against susceptible bacteria. However, allergic reactions have been reported with all cephalosporins, including second-generation cephalosporins, and symptoms may include a rash, hives (urticaria), swelling, or rarely, anaphylaxis

Examples - cefoxitin, cefuroxime

8. Third generation cephalosporins?

Ans) Third-generation cephalosporins are a group of broad-spectrum antibiotics that can get rid of gram-positive and gram-negative bacteria. These types of antibiotics are bactericidal by interrupting their cell wall.

Uses

- Bone and joint infections
- Lower respiratory tract infections
- Urinary tract infections
- Central nervous system infections
- Gynaecological infections
- Intra-abdominal infections
- Skin infections

Adverse drug reactions
Urticaria, Skin rashes & swellings rarely anaphylaxis

9. Pharmacological basis for combining beta lactamase inhibitors with beta lactam antibiotics?

Ans) The enzyme beta lactamase can destroy the beta lactam antibiotics. So, by using the beta lactamase inhibitors like clavulanic acid, Sulbactam when combined with beta lactam anti-biotics like ampicillin and cefoperazone can increase its effectiveness

10. What is anti-pseudomonal penicillin?

    Ans) Penicillin like piperacillin, Ticarcillin which have activity of penicillin and aminopenicillin which can be used against pseudomonas, klebsiella and enterococcus

11. Why imipenem and Cilastatin combined preparation used for hospital acquired infection?

    Ans) It is because of the beneficial interaction, by inhibiting the dihydropeptidase -1 on the brush border cells of the renal tubules Cilastatin inhibits the rapid metabolism of the Imipenam.

12. Pseudomembranous enterocolitis?

    Ans) Metronidazole and Vancomycin are the DOC. Sometimes penicillin such as Amoxicillin and Ampicillin are also used.

13. Treatment of UTI in pregnancy?

    Ans) For symptomatic UTI, Amoxicillin 500 mg tid for 3 days as empirical therapy. Modifications are done according to urine culture after 7 days. Fluoroquinolones should not be used in pregnancy.

14. Enumerate the antibiotics which act by inhibiting cell wall synthesis?

    Ans)

    - Beta lactam antibiotics e.g., Penicillin, Ceftriaxone
    - Glycopeptide antibiotics e.g., Vancomycin, Bleomycin

15. Name 2 Bactericidal and Bacteriostatic antibiotics?

    Ans) Aminoglycosides like Gentamicin, Tobramycin -Bactericidal
    Beta lactam antibiotics like Amoxicillin and Cefazolin - Bactericidal
    Tetracyclines,macrolides are Bacteriostatic

∙ ∙ ∙

TETRACYCLINE AND CHLORAMPHENICOL

1. Classification of Tetracyclines

   Ans)

   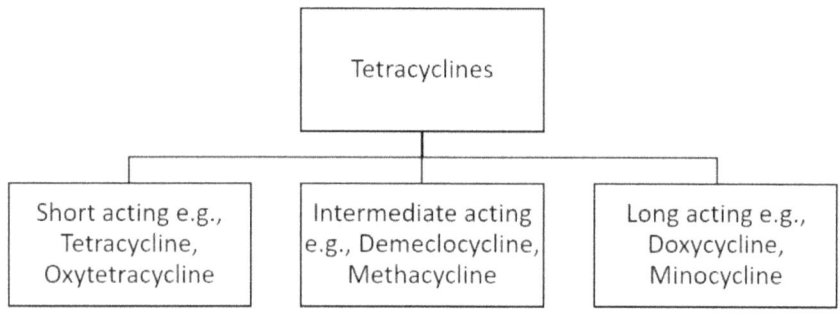

   Classification of tetracyclines

2. Chloramphenicol or Ceftriaxone in typhoid fever?

   Ans) Ceftriaxone due to its higher sensitivity to salmonella species.

3. Mention differences between tetracycline and doxycycline?

   Ans)

- Tetracycline can affect all the beneficial bacteria that make up the gut microbiome and can cause diarrhoea, whereas doxycycline doesn't affect the gut microbiome
- Tetracycline aggravates preexisting renal failure whereas doxycycline doesn't
- Doxycycline is highly potent than tetracycline and have longer plasma half-life

- Tetracycline is excreted through kidney whereas doxycycline through liver so that doxycycline can be given to patients with renal failure

4. Comment on the usage of tetracycline in pregnancy?

Ans) Tetracycline is generally not used in pregnancy due to its teratogenic effects.

• • •

AMINO GLYCOSIDES

1. Aminoglycosides?

Ans) Examples – Streptomycin, Neomycin, Tobramycin, Amikacin
Mechanism of action - By blocking the 30S ribosomal subunit of microbials except for Streptomycin which blocks the 50S ribosomal subunit.

<u>Common properties</u>

- They cause ototoxicity and nephrotoxicity
- They exhibit partial cross resistance among themselves
- They are not metabolized in our body and are excreted unchanged in urine
- Distributed mainly in the extracellular fluid and poorly penetrates into the CSF
- Bactericidal on gram negative anaerobes, more active in alkaline pH

<u>Adverse effects</u>
Ototoxicity, Nephrotoxicity and rarely neuromuscular blockade and hypersensitivity reactions

• • •

SULPHONAMIDES

1. Cotrimoxazole?

Ans) It is a WHO approved fixed dose combination which consists of sulphamethoxazole and trimethoprim in a 5:1 combination which gives a supra-additive effect by sequential blockage of the synthesis of folic acid. Even though individually both causes a bacteriostatic effect in combination it causes bactericidal effect, it also reduces the formation of resistance. Here the Sulphamethoxazole inhibits the dihydrofolate synthetase enzyme whereas trimethoprim blocks the dihydrofolate reductase enzyme.

Pharmacokinetics – It is well absorbed orally and excreted through urine. Well tolerated

Uses – To treat urinary tract infection, pneumocystis jiroveci infection, Respiratory tract infection and bacterial diarrhoeas.

• • •

MACROLIDE AND OTHER ANTIBACTERIALS

1. Mechanism of action of macrolides?

Ans) They prevents the Protein synthesis machinery of the bacteria by preventing the 50S ribosomal subunit. It is usually bacteriostatic but can be bactericidal in high concentrations. Increased action in alkaline pH

2. Clarithromycin?

Ans) Clarithromycin is a semi-synthetic macrolide. So as other macrolides its mechanism of action is by inhibiting the 50S ribosomal subunit of the bacteria and inhibit their protein synthesis, so that it is mainly bacteriostatic but can be bactericidal at higher concentrations. It is having a wide antibiotic spectrum which includes the mycobacterium leprae, mycobacterium avium complex it is there in triple regimen of H. pylori infection.

3. Enumerate macrolide antibiotics and mention its 4 uses?

Ans) Erythromycin, Clarithromycin, Azithromycin
Uses

- To treat atypical community acquired pneumonia
- As a component of the triple regimen to treat H. pylori infection
- To treat acute non-specific urethritis
- To treat chlamydidiasis

4. Specify the important spectrum of vancomycin?

Ans) To treat serious staphylococcal infections like MRSA. Staphylococci, Streptococci, Enterococci, Diphtheroids, Clostridium species.

5. Linezolid?

Ans) Linezolid is a synthetic oxazolidinone antimicrobial drug. It is a high-end reserve antibiotic used to treat vancomycin resistant enterococcal infections, infections complicated by bacteraemia, bacterial pneumonia. Adverse effects - Nausea, Vomiting, Diarrhoea and Head ache

6. Uses and adr of vancomycin?

Ans) Uses

- To treat intestinal infections caused by Clostridium difficile.
- To treat severe bacterial infections which are resistant to other drugs

Adverse reactions

- Allergic reactions, Nephrotoxicity, Ototoxicity, Redman's syndrome (Patient reaches a shock like state after rapid i.v. infusion)

7. Azithromycin?

Ans) Azithromycin is a macrolide antibiotic that fights bacteria. It's used to treat many different types of infections caused by bacteria, such as respiratory infections, skin infections, ear infections, eye infections, and sexually transmitted diseases. Administered orally or intra venously. Given 1 hour before or 2 hours after food. More active against H.Influenzae than erythromycin and Clarithromycin. It is well absorbed, wide tissue didtribution, Long acting (Once daily use)

Mechanism of action – (Same as macrolides)

Contra indications- liver diseases, kidney diseases, myasthenia gravis, a heart rhythm disorder, low levels of potassium in your blood, or long QT syndrome.

Common side effects of Azithromycin include nausea, abdominal pain, and diarrhoea.

8. What are streptogramins and mention one use of it?

Ans) Streptogramins are a class of antibiotics used to treat methicillin resistant staphylococcus aureus and some vancomycin resistant enterococcus.

• • •

Anti-tuberculosis drugs

1. Treatment regimen of drug sensitive tuberculosis?

Ans) According to RNTCP 2016 guidelines

- For new patients which means those tuberculosis patients who have either not taken anti-tuberculosis drugs or taken them for less than 1 month
- In the intensive phase of first 2 months Isoniazid, Rifampicin, Pyrazinamide, Ethambutol (HRZE) are given, and for the next four months of continuous phase Isoniazid, Rifampicin and Ethambutol are given
- For previously treated tuberculosis cases which means those tuberculosis patients who have taken anti-tuberculosis drugs for more than 1 month. This includes tuberculosis patients who have lost follow up, treatment failure cases and recurrent tb cases
- In the in the intensive phase of 3 months first 2 months are given with Isoniazid, Rifampicin, Pyrazinamide, Ethambutol and Streptomycin

(HRZES) and the next one-month streptomycin is avoided (HRZE) and in the continuous phase of next 5 months Isoniazid, Rifampicin and Ethambutol are given (HRE)
- The drugs are given through directly observed short-course therapy (DOTS) to ensure that the drug is being consumed.

Mnemonic – Pyrazinamide similar to pyros(fire) burns out in the intensive phase not used in continuous phase. Streptomycin (S is like 2) uses only in the first 2 months that also when the patient comes second time (Previously treated cases) also in previously treated cases intensive phase is 3 months and it doesn't use in the 3rd month.

2. Treatment of multi drug resistant tuberculosis?

Ans) Multi drug resistant tuberculosis means development of resistance against at least any two of the first line anti-tuberculosis drugs, sometimes resistance to the first line anti tb drug Rifampicin itself may be considered as multi drug resistant tb since it is the major drug with sterilizing activity. The treatment consists of at least four drugs which are sensitive according to the anti-microbial sensitivity testing. To prevent the neurotoxicity due to some of the drugs like ethionamide and cycloserine, pyridoxine should be administered. The strategy that we follows is DOTS-Plus strategy.

The drugs used to treat the intensive phase which is about 6 to 9 months is Kanamycin, Ethambutol, Ethionamide, Pyrazinamide, Cycloserine, Levofloxacin (Mnemonic-KEEP in CaLl intensively)

The drugs used to treat the continuous phase which is about 18 months is Cycloserine, Ethionamide, Ethambutol, Levofloxacin (CEEL (Seal) it properly in continuous phase.

3. Treatment of tuberculosis in pregnant ladies?

Ans) Similar as others except

- Streptomycin is not given
- Pyridoxine is given

After ruling out active TB the baby should be given 6 months of isoniazid preventive therapy, followed by BCG vaccination. Breast feeding shouldn't

be discouraged.
   If MDR-TB
   If the lady is less than 20 weeks pregnant Advice MTP

- If MTP is done – Then start or continue the treatment
- If MTP is not done – If less than 12 weeks omit Kanamycin and Ethionamide and add para-amino salicylic acid

If greater than 12 weeks omit Kanamycin only and add para-amino salicylic acid and continue it till delivery. Replace para-amino salicylic acid with Kanamycin after delivery.

4. Rifampicin – Mechanism of action, Uses, Adverse effects?

Ans) Given orally, well absorbed in g.i.t but food might decrease the absorption, metabolised in liver, undergoes enterohepatic recycling and then gets excreted in Urine. Acts as a sterilizing agent.
   Mechanism of action
   It binds to the DNA-dependent RNA polymerase and prevents the RNA synthesis of the mycobacteria.
   Uses

- To treat and for the prophylaxis of tuberculosis
- To treat leprosy
- As adjuvant to treat staphylococcal infections
- To treat Brucellosis by combining with doxycycline
- For the prophylaxis of meningitis occurring due to H. Influenza or meningococci

Adverse effects

- Hepatitis
- Staining of body fluids like urine, sweat, tears, sputum etc. which is harmless but prior informing to the patients is required to prevent panicking
- Gastrointestinal disturbances like nausea, vomiting
- Musculoskeletal pain, fever, chills, headache

5. Rifampicin in a patient on oral contraceptives?

Ans) Being an enzyme inducer Rifampicin increases the metabolism of the oral contraceptives and may lead to contraceptive failure so that a patient on oral contraceptives should be turn to other contraceptive methods like barrier method before starting of tuberculosis therapy.

6. Mechanism of action and adverse drug reactions of other first line anti-tuberculosis drugs?

Ans)

Drug	Mechanism of action	Adverse drug reaction
Isoniazid	It blocks the mycolic acid synthesis in mycobacteria by entering the mycobacteria which converts it into reactive metabolite with the help of a catalase-peroxidase enzyme which forms an adduct which inhibits the InhA and KasA gene required for mycolic acid synthesis, also with NADP which is required for DHFRase for DNA synthesis	Peripheral neuritis, Hepatitis
Pyrazinamide	Inhibits the mycolic acid synthesis by the active metabolite pyrazinoic acid	Hepatotoxicity and hyper uricemia
Ethambutol	Inhibition of arabinosyl transferases which causes the inhibition of arabinoglycan synthesis which is required for the incorporation of mycolic acid to mycobacterial cell wall	E for eye. Causes retrobulbar neuritis
Streptomycin	By binding to the 30S ribosomal subunit	Hypersensitivity reactions

Table - Anti tb drugs

7. Treatment of MAC?

Ans) A regimen consisting of macrolides (clarithromycin or azithromycin) with rifampin and ethambutol has been recommended; this regimen significantly improves the treatment of MAC pulmonary disease and should be maintained for at least 12 months after negative sputum culture conversion.

• • •

ANTI LEPROTICS

1. 2 uses and adverse drug reactions of Clofazimine?

   Ans)

Uses	Adverse drug reactions
To treat Parkinson's disease To treat Hyperprolactinemia	Dry skin Change in skin colour

   Uses and adr of Clofazimine

2. Treatment of leprosy?

   Ans) First determine whether it is paucibacillary leprosy or multibacillary leprosy. Paucibacillary means less than or equal to 5 skin lesions and multibacillary means more than 5 skin lesions.
   For paucibacillary leprosy Rifampicin 600 mg once monthly is given under supervision and Dapsone is self-administered 100 mg daily for 6 months.
   For multibacillary leprosy Rifampicin 600mg once monthly and Clofazimine 300 mg once monthly is given under supervision and Dapsone 100 mg and Clofazimine 50 mg are self-administered daily for 1 year.

3. Lepra reaction?

   Ans) There are 2 types of lepra reaction lepra 1 reaction (Reversal reaction) which is a type 4 hypersensitivity reaction and lepra 2 reaction (Erythema nodosum leprosum) which is a type 3 hypersensitivity reaction (Mnemonic- 1+4 =2+3)
   Type 1 reaction – drug used is prednisolone or clofazimine
   Type 2 reaction - drug used are prednisolone, clofazimine, aspirin and chloroquine.

Severe form of type 2 reaction is treated with Thalidomide (Except in pregnancy)

Thalidomide is used since it blocks the selective gene expression of tumour necrosis factor-α involved in the pathogenesis of nerve damage in leprosy and other mechanisms contributing to its anti-inflammatory effect.

4. Intermittent ROM regimen?

Ans) It includes Rifampicin(600mg), Ofloxacin(400mg) and Minocycline(100mg) once a month to treat leprosy. 3-6 months for paucibacillary and 12 to 24 months for multi bacillary leprosy.

• • •

ANTI-FUNGALS

1. Griseofulvin?

Ans) Griseofulvin is an anti-fungal drug which can be used to treat infections caused by dermatophytes

Mechanism of action – It interacts with the polymerized microtubules and disrupts the mitotic spindle, thus griseofulvin acts as a spindle poison and inhibits the fungal growth by being a fungistatic.

Pharmacokinetics – Griseofulvin is highly bioavailable through oral route so can be administered orally. The bio-availability is further increased by consuming it along with fatty food.

Drug interactions – It is an enzyme inducer and it reduces the effectiveness of warfarin therapy and causes failure of oral contraceptives

Adverse drug reactions – Insomnia, Dizziness, Rash, Numbness or tingling in hands or feet, Headache, Tiredness and dizziness

2. Griseofulvin or Miconazole to treat candidiasis?

Ans) Miconazole because of its targeted action of fungus like candida, and unlike griseofulvin which causes systemic side effects it only causes local side effects.

3. Fluconazole or Ketoconazole in fungal meningitis?

Ans) Fluconazole due to its increased effectiveness and decreased side effects

4. Two differences between Fluconazole and Ketoconazole?

Ans) Spectrum of activity – Fluconazole is more effective against candida albicans and cryptococcus whereas Ketoconazole against tinea species, blastomycosis etc.
Side effects and drug interactions – Fluconazole is having lesser side effects and drug interactions than that of ketoconazole. Fluconazole doesn't inhibit the synthesis of steroids and doesn't have antiandrogenic effect

5. Fluconazole?

Ans) Fluconazole is a drug which comes under azole group of antifungals among it under triazole category. Mechanism of action is believed to be by blocking the synthesis of fungal cell membrane. It has high oral bioavailability. It is used to treat candidiasis, and meningitis (cryptococcal and coccidiodal). The reason for usage of it in meningitis is due to its ability to freely cross the blood brain barrier. The adverse effects caused due to it are nausea, vomiting, abdominal discomfort and diarrhoea

6. Itraconazole?

Ans) Group of drugs – Triazole
Mechanism of action – By blocking the 14-α demethylase of the fungus thereby preventing the formation of ergosterol which is required for the cell membrane formation of the fungus
Pharmacokinetics – Metabolism happens at the liver, High plasma binding
Drug interactions – Due to its microsomal enzyme inducer property
Uses – To treat Aspergillosis, Blastomycosis, Sporotrichosis, Histoplasmosis
Adverse drug reactions – Head ache, Dizziness, Drowsiness and Tiredness

7. Amphotericin B?

Ans) It is a broad spectrum anti-fungal drug
Class of drug – Polyene class of antifungals
Mechanism of action – Tightly binds to the ergosterol of the fungal cell membrane and forms pores and channels in the membrane which increases the permeability of the membrane and causes the leakage of intracellular contents and there by death of the fungi.
Pharmacokinetics – Highly bound to plasma proteins and tissues. It is unable to cross the blood brain barrier. Metabolism happens in the liver and excreted through bile and urine. Not absorbed well from gut, not effective orally.
Uses – To treat Aspergillosis, Mucormycosis, Sporotrichosis, Cryptococcosis, Histoplasmosis. (Systemic mycoses)
Adverse drug reactions – Nephrotoxicity, Anaemia, Electrolyte disturbances, Fever, Chills, Dyspnoea, Headache

8. Drugs used to treat onychomycosis?

Ans) Triazoles and Terbinafine.

• • •

ANTI-VIRAL DRUGS

1. Oseltamivir?

Ans) Oseltamivir is an antiviral drug of class neuraminidase inhibitors,
Mechanism of action – By inhibiting the neuraminidase of the virus thereby inhibits the release of the influenza virus from the infected cells
Pharmacokinetics – It is highly bioavailable and excreted mainly through the liver
Use - To treat influenza A and influenza B.
Adverse drug reactions – Vomiting, Diarrhoea, Abdominal pain, Bronchitis, dizziness, Fatigue and headache.

2. Protease inhibitors?

Ans) These are a group of anti-retro viral drugs.

Mechanism of action – By preventing the cleavage of viral proteins by the HIV proteases and thereby causing the production of immature non-infectious viral particles and thereby preventing the transmission to other cells

Cross resistance is common

Pharmacokinetics – Metabolism takes place in the liver.

Adverse drug reactions – Nausea, Vomiting, Diarrhoea, Kidney stones are seen with Indinavir

Examples – Indinavir, Ritonavir

Ritonavir boosting – Ritonavir being a microsomal enzyme inhibitor increases the bioavailability of other protease inhibitors when taken along with low dose ritonavir by increasing the half-life of them.

3. Interferon α?

Ans) Interferon α is one type among the three types of interferons. Interferons are basically proteins with anti-viral property produced by the virus infected cells and it can also be produced by recombinant DNA technology.

Mechanism of action – They inhibits almost every step in the pathogenesis of the virus beginning with the viral penetration, transcription of the viral mRNA, translation of the mRNA and the assembly and release of the viral proteins.

Uses – For treatment of genital warts, hepatitis B, hepatitis C. In immunocompromised people to treat Kaposi sarcoma and herpetic infections.

Adverse effects – Bone-marrow suppression, Thyroid dysfunction, Alopecia, Myalgia, Fever, Head-ache

4. Mechanism of action of Acyclovir?

Ans) Due to the ability of the herpetic virus to code for a viral thymidine kinase capable of phosphorylating acyclovir to a monophosphate acyclovir it is selectively taken up by the herpetic viruses and then with the help of cellular enzymes it is then converted to acyclovir diphosphate and triphosphate which inhibits the viral DNA synthesis and its replication.

• • •

ANTI-MALARIAL DRUGS

1. Classify antimalarial drugs?

   Ans)

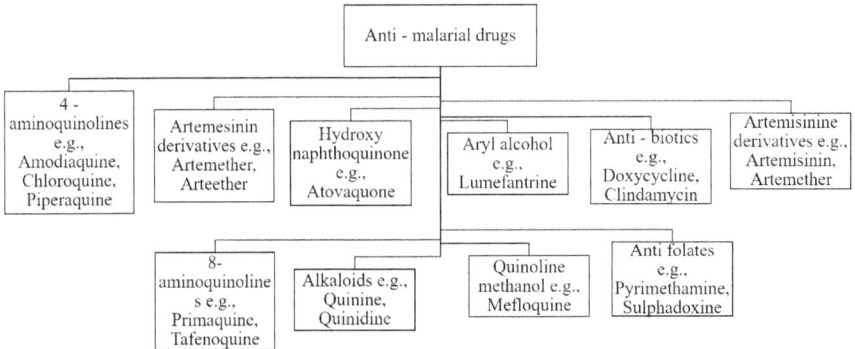

Classification of anti-malarials

Also, antibiotics like Doxycycline and clindamycin are also used

(Mnemonics – A queen (4-aminoqinolines) with 8 other queens (8-aminoquinolines) in the Art gallery (Artemisinin derivatives) was taking water and naastha (Hydroxy naphthoquinone) (water -hydroxy, naastha- breakfast in hindi) at that time one of the queens was alcoholic (Alkaloids examples also queen- quinine and quinidine) she threw away the flowers on the dining table (Antifolates -Remember as anti-flowers) and asked are you alcoholic? (Aryl alcohols) and fell into queens metheck (Meth means body in Malayalam) fell and told I came in a flow (Quinoline methanol - Mefloquine))

2. Explain the mechanism of action, adverse effects and dose of Chloroquine?

   Ans) Chloroquine being basic accumulates in the acidic food vacuole of the malarial parasites and blocks the conversion of the heme to hemozoin by forming a complex with the heme. Heme being toxic to the parasite kills the parasite

3. Sulphadoxine and pyrimethamine in malarial treatment?

Ans) They are antifolates used to prevent serious malaria when other medicines do not work. It exhibits synergistic effect to kill the malarial parasite by sequential blockade of the folic acid synthesis. When Sulphadoxine blocks the dihydropteroate synthase, pyrimethamine inhibits dihydrofolate reductase.

4. Artemisinin based combination therapy (ACT) in malaria?

Ans) Artemisinin can kill 90-95% of the malarial parasites but have short half-life so rapidly develops resistance so that artemisinin is always given as a combination to treat malaria.
ACT regimes for the treatment of falciparum malaria. 4 ACT regimes are currently recommended by WHO

- Artesunate + Mefloquine
- Artesunate + Sulphadoxine + Pyrimethamine (Other states)
- Artesunate + Amodiaquine
- Artemether + Lumefantrine (North eastern states)

5. Radical cure in plasmodium vivax infection?

Ans) Primaquine 15mg daily for 14 days simultaneously or after chloroquine or other schizonticides reduces the relapse rate.
In glucose -6- phosphate deficient peoples caution is taken and 0.75mg/Kg once a week is given for 8 weeks

6. Treatment of severe and complicated falciparum malaria?

Ans) According to guidelines for treatment of malaria, 3rd edition; WHO 2015

- Artesunate 2.4 mg/Kg stat is given intravenously or intramuscularly followed by 2.4mg/Kg after 12 and 24 hours, and then once in a day for

1 week, When the patient can take oral medication switch over to ACT regimen 3 day orally Or
- Artemether 3.2 mg/Kg on first day followed by 1.6mg/Kg daily for 1 week, When the patient can take oral medication switch over to ACT regimen 3 day orally

7. Mention the adverse effects and therapeutic uses of chloroquine?

   Ans) Therapeutic uses
   Mnemonic – MALARIA G
   M – To treat malaria
   A – To treat amoebic liver abscess
   L – To treat Lepra reaction
   A – To treat atopic dermatitis
   R – Rheumatoid arthritis
   I – Infectious mononucleosis
   A – Autoimmune disorders like systemic lupus erythematosus
   G – Giardiasis
   Adverse effects

- Gastro intestinal side effects – Nausea, Vomiting
- CNS side effects - Headache and visual disturbances, Convulsions
- CVS side effects – Cardiac arrest, Cardiac arrhythmias

8. Uses and adverse effects of diethyl carbamazine citrate?

   Ans) Uses

- To treat lymphatic filariasis, to treat pulmonary eosinophilia, to treat loiasis.

   Adverse drug reactions

- Fever, Skin rash, Joint pain, Muscle pain

9. List two drugs for the chemoprophylaxis of malaria?

   Ans) Chloroquine phosphate, Mefloquine

10. Pseudomembranous enterocolitis?

Ans) Metronidazole and Vancomycin are the DOC. Sometimes penicillin such as Amoxicillin and Ampicillin are also used.

• • •

ANTI-AMOEBIC DRUGS

1. Metronidazole?

Ans) Class of drug – Nitroimidazole
Mechanism of action – The highly reactive nitro radical produced by the drug by accepting electrons from the ferredoxins damages the DNA of the microorganism and causes its death
Pharmacokinetics – Absorption happens through the small intestine and excretion through the liver
Uses – To treat Entamoeba histolytica infection, to treat Giardiasis, to treat trichomonas Vaginalis infection and for the extraction of Guinea worm. (Mnemonic – VEGetarian foods will Get in the metro)
Adverse drug reactions – Gastro intestinal side effects; Nausea, Dry mouth and metallic taste
Central nervous system side effects; Dizziness, Headache, Vertigo, Irritability, Disulfiram like actions

2. Metronidazole and ceftriaxone for brain abscess?

Ans) To treat brain abscess a combination of metronidazole and ceftriaxone is used. Ceftriaxone is used for coverage against streptococci, Enterobacteriaceae and most common anaerobes whereas metronidazole is selected for its efficacy against bacteroides fragilis.

3. Metronidazole and diloxanide furoate in Intestinal amoebiasis?

Ans) They causes beneficial effects. Metronidazole being a tissue amoebicide and diloxanide furoate a luminal amoebicide it provides a complete cure.

ANTHELMINTIC DRUGS

1. Albendazole?

   Ans) Class of drug – Benzimidazole
   Pharmacokinetics – Can be taken orally. Like Griseofulvin its absorption is also increases when taken along with fatty food. Metabolism happens in the liver.
   Mechanism of action – Inhibits the polymerization of β tubulin into microtubules followed by inhibition of glucose uptake and transport.
   Dosage – 400 mg single dose for adults and children above 2 years of age and 200 mg single dose for children between 1 and 2 years of age.
   Uses – To treat Neurocysticercosis, to treat nematode infections such as of Pi worm, round worm, Hook worm, Thread worm, to treat Hydatid disease, to treat filariasis

2. Ivermectin?

   Ans) Ivermectin is an anthelminthic.
   Mechanism of action – Ivermectin binds to the glutamate-activated chloride channels existing in the nerve or muscle cells of nematode with a specific and high affinity, causing hyperpolarization of nerve or muscle cells by increasing permeability of chloride ion through the cell membrane, and as a result the parasites are paralyzed to death.
   Pharmacokinetics – Good oral absorption and mechanism happens in the liver
   Uses – To treat Onchocerciasis, Strongyloidiasis, Ascariasis, Cutaneous larva migrans, filariasis, gnathostomiasis, trichuriasis.

CHAPTER XI

Gastro intestinal drugs

PEPTIC ULCER AND GASTRO ESOPHAGEAL REFLUX DISEASE

1. Classification of drugs used in peptic ulcer?

   Ans)

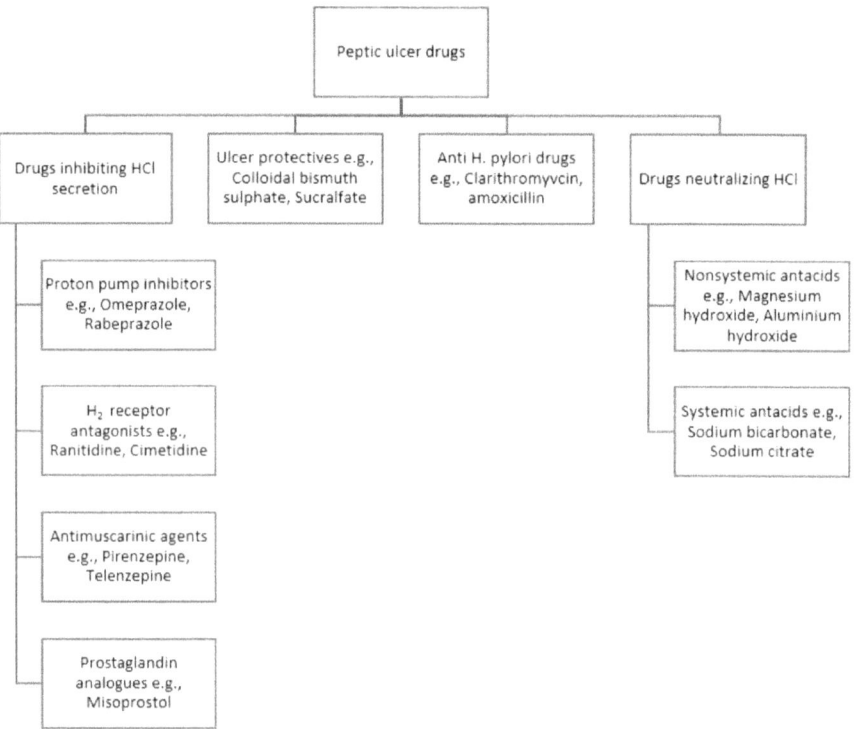

Classification of drugs for peptic ulcer

2. NSAID induced peptic ulcer?

Ans) Proton pump inhibitors are drug of choice. H2 receptor antagonists and prostaglandins are also used.

3. Ranitidine?

Ans) It is a nonimidazole H2 blocker which reduces the HCl secretion used to treat gastric ulcer.
It has additional benefits from that of Cimetidine

- Lower side effects, Lower interactions with other drugs
- No CNS effects
- Antiandrogenic effects are less, so preferred over Cimetidine in males

4. Proton pump inhibitors?

Ans) Examples – Omeprazole, Rabeprazole
Omeprazole is a proton pump inhibitor which inhibits the gastric acid secretion. Other examples Rabeprazole and Lansoprazole
Mechanism of action – Omeprazole as well as all other proton pump after getting absorbed in the small intestine gets diffused into the parietal cell through the blood then at the acidic p^H of the canaliculi of the parietal cell it gets converted into the active charged form sulphenamide and bind covalently to the SH group of the proton pump to inactivate it irreversibly

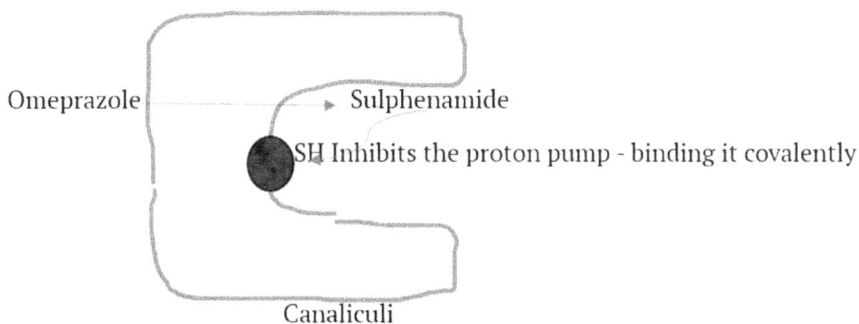

Mechanism of action of proton pumps

- Pharmacokinetics – Good oral absorption. Food inhibits its absorption.
- Drug interactions – Omeprazole should not be given with itraconazole because omeprazole affects the kinetics of itraconazole which leads to a reduction of its bioavailability and Cmax. So, these 2 drugs should not be used together.
- Uses – To treat Peptic ulcer, Gastroesophageal reflux disease, Zollinger-Ellison syndrome and to reduce the risk of aspiration pneumonia.
- Adverse drug reactions – Diarrhoea, Headache, Nausea, Abdominal pain.
- Drug interactions – Omeprazole decreases the bioavailability of Itraconazole by altering its kinetics

5. Ulcer protective agents?

   Ans) Examples – Sucralfate, Colloidal bismuth sulphate
   <u>Mechanism of action</u>

- It forms a sticky polymer which adheres to the ulcer base in the acidic environment of stomach and protects it.
- Produces a cytoprotective effect by stimulating the release of epidermal growth factor and prostaglandins locally
- Enhances the mucosal defence and repair by increasing the mucus and bicarbonate secretion

   Uses – To treat gastric ulcer, Oesophagitis, Gastroesophageal reflux disease, Rectal ulcer
   Adverse drug reactions – Constipation

6. Triple drug regimen of H. pylori infection?

   Ans) Mnemonic – Patient in the hall (H. pylori) should **call** 3 times to get the medicines, only if 500 times called morning and evening at least 30 people land. A for 1 – 1st letter of alphabet
   C – Clarithromycin 500 mg twice daily
   A - Amoxicillin 1 g twice daily

L - Lansoprazole 30 mg twice daily

7. Non-systemic antacids?

Ans) These are antacids which does not get absorbed into the systemic circulation and cause systemic alkalosis. For example, Aluminium hydroxide, Magnesium hydroxide, Magnesium trisilicate, Calcium carbonate.

Mechanism of action – By reacting with the acid in the stomach the it reacts with the HCl in the stomach to get converted into its chloride salt and water and the chloride salt reacts with bicarbonate in the stomach so, bicarbonates are not available for systemic absorption and thereby no systemic alkalosis.

The Aluminium hydroxide and magnesium hydroxide are given together because

- Being a rapid onset drug magnesium hydroxide, its effect is not sustained and being a slow onset drug aluminium hydroxide doesn't give a rapid action so by combining them a rapid sustained effect is obtained.

- The aluminium ions relax the smooth muscles and prolongs the gastric emptying time and causes constipation whereas the magnesium hydroxide by increasing the osmolarity causes increased absorption of water from outside and causes mild diarrhoea and when these two are used together they gets cancelled each other.
- The individual doses and thereby systemic toxicity can be reduced.

8. Prostaglandins in peptic ulcer?

Ans) Prostaglandin analogues like Misoprostol are used to treat gastric ulcer because it inhibits the gastric acid secretion, increases the mucosal blood flow and increases mucus and bicarbonate secretion.

9. Name two H2 antihistaminic?

Ans) Cimetidine, Ranitidine

10. Name two laxatives?

Ans) Bisacodyl and lactulose

∙ ∙ ∙

ANTI EMETICS

1. Classification of antiemetics?

   Ans)

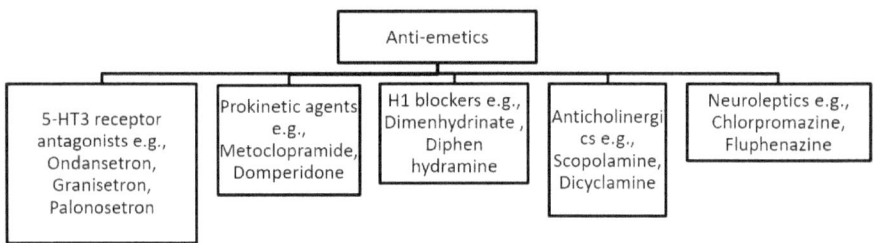

Classification of anti-emetics

2. Ondansetron?

   Ans) Ondansetron is an anti-emetic drug in the drug class 5-HT_3-Receptor antagonists.
   Mechanism of action – It is having both central action and peripheral action.
   Central action – In the Creutzfeldt nucleus (CTZ) and solitary tract nucleus it blocks the 5-HT_3 receptors.
   Peripheral action – By blocking the 5-HT_3 receptors on the vagal afferents in the gut. Since in case of chemotherapy the reason for the vomiting is the impulses got to the Creutzfeldt nucleus and solitary tract nucleus from the vagal afferents in the gut through the 5-HT released from the enterochromaffin cells of the intestinal mucosa due to the tissue damages caused in the stomach due to the anticancer therapies, the peripheral action of these drug makes it possible to use in the vomiting

caused due to the cancer therapy (Normally due to the longest duration of action among the 5-HT_3 receptor antagonists Palonosetron is used for cancer treatment induced vomiting, Granisetron transdermal patches are also used)

Uses

- To treat chemotherapy induced vomiting
- To treat irritable bowel syndrome
- To treat hyperemesis gravidarum

Adverse effects - Diarrhoea, Dizziness, Headache

3. Metoclopramide? Or Cisapride?

Ans) (Mnemonic to study both metoclopramide action and Ondansetron action- Oh! MD is coming. Ondansetron only in the 5-HT_3 receptors and metoclopramide also in the D_2 receptors at 3 sites upper GIT and CTZ which is at the blood brain barrier and in the basal ganglia and also the 5-HT_3 and 5-HT_4 in the stomach. Its normal action is blocking the receptor but fearing the elder brother 5-HT_4 it stimulates it, to inhibit the 5-HT_3 it needs in high concentration as there is need to check whether elder brother is coming)

It comes under the class of prokinetic agents.

Pharmacokinetics – High oral bioavailability, poorly binds the plasma proteins and crosses the blood brain barrier.

Drug interactions – Competes with levodopa for D_2 binding site. So, not given in levodopa induced vomiting.

Mechanism of action

- By blocking the D_2 receptors in the upper gastro intestinal system it promotes the cholinergic stimulation of the gastrointestinal smooth muscles by removing its inhibitory effect, it causes increased peristalsis.
- By blocking the D_2 receptors in the Creutzfeldt nucleus it causes its antiemetic effect.
- By stimulating the 5-HT_4 interneurons in the gut it increases the release of acetyl choline from the myenteric motor neurons by increasing acetylcholine activity.
- By blocking the 5-HT_3 receptors in the myenteric interneurons in the GIT it increases the acetylcholine release and causes anti-emetic effects.

Adverse effects – It causes drowsiness, diarrhoea and dizziness

4. Why domperidone is preferred over metoprolol in children?

Ans) Because metoclopramide has extra pyramidal effects and can cause muscle dystonia in children.

5. Aprepitant?

Ans) It is an antiemetic of the group Neurokinin receptor antagonist.
<u>Mechanism of action</u> – Being a highly selective competitive antagonist of the G-protein coupled neurokinin-1 receptor which are present in both central and peripheral nervous system and throughout the gastro intestinal tract, it blocks the substance P which is a nociceptive neurotransmitter. By blocking the NK-1 receptors at nucleus tractus solitarius and area postrema which plays critical roles in the vomiting reflex it blocks the vomiting also the binding of NK-1 receptors throughout the GIT aids in its anti-emetic effect

Pharmacokinetics

- Absorption - Absorption decreases with increasing dose
- Distribution – High plasma protein binding and high volume of distribution
- Metabolism – Metabolism happens in the liver
- Excretion – 50% through urine and 50% through faeces.

• • •

CONSTIPATION AND DIARRHOEA

1. Super ORS?

Ans) Addition to the normal ORS it contains lysine or glycine which is an essential amino-acid which enhances the absorption of sodium and water from the lumen of gut along with it also induces the reabsorption of endogenous intestinal secretion thereby reducing the volume, frequency and duration of diarrhoea.

2. Lactulose?

Ans) It is a semi-synthetic disachharide which can't be absorbed or digested in the intestine so it retains water and and act as an osmotic purgative. The breakdown products of the Lactulose are acidic which causes reduction in PH and an unfavorable situation for the ammonia producing bacterias, so used in hepatic coma.

CHAPTER XII

Hormones and related drugs

Thyroid

1. Radioactive Iodine?

   Ans) Normally I131 isotope of iodine is used for the treatment of hyperthyroidism. The radioactive iodine is also taken up by the thyroid gland which undergoes radioactive decay there to get Ý rays and β particles among it the β particles causes the destruction of the follicular cells which was producing the thyroid hormone and causes its fibrosis and thereby it corrects the hyperthyroidism.
   Route of administration - Oral administration in the form of capsules or solution.
   Uses – For the treatment of Graves's disease, Toxic nodular goitre in the elderly patients, For the treatment of hyperthyroidism when the preferred surgery cannot be done.
   Adverse drug reactions – Hypothyroidism
   Contra indications – Pregnancy due to the increased risk of getting cancer to the child in future.

2. Drugs that can be administered hyperthyroidism caused due to TSH suppression?

   Ans) Thioamide derivatives like Carbimazole and Methimazole.

3. What is the mechanism of action of thioamide derivatives?

   Ans) They act mainly by inhibiting the activity of thyroid peroxidase enzyme which causes the blockage of thyroid hormone synthesis at 3 steps, In the conversion of iodide to iodine, the iodination of tyrosine residues in the thyroglobulin and the coupling reaction of mono-iodotyronine to di-iodotyronine

4. What is the use of propranolol in the treatment of thyroid storm?

   Ans) Propranolol is the preferred beta blocker in the treatment of thyroid storm due to its additional effect of blocking the peripheral conversion of inactive T4 to active T3 form along with reducing the symptoms of thyrotoxicosis like palpitation, tachycardia and tremors.

5. Which all anti-thyroid drugs are preferred during pregnancy?

   Ans) Thioamides among it propylthiouracil (Mnemonics - note Thai (Mother in Tamil) for remembering thioamides in pregnancy). Other examples – Carbimazole, Methimazole

6. Thyrotoxic crisis?

   Ans) Assume that Siddhu's mother in the crisis by a disease. Then we are telling Siddhu "Hospitalise and give support properly to the mother, Siddhu"
   H – Hospitalise the patient
   Supportive care – Since in thyrotoxic crisis high temperature cool it using cooling blankets, sedation etc.
   Properly – Give propranolol
   Mother – thai – Propylthiouracil (Preferred drug in pregnancy)
   Si – Sodium ipodate
   dd -we only need 1 d delete other – Diltiazem
   hu – Hydrocortisone (U for to reach ullil(inside) rapidly give through intravenous route)

7. Management of Myxoedema coma?

   Ans) For hypothyroidism – Large initial dose of 300-500 μg T4, if no response adds T3

   - For hypocortisolaemia iv hydrocortisone 200-400mg
   - Provide ventilation

- Give blankets for hypothermia, no active rewarming
- For hyponatremia – mild fluid restriction
- Hypotension – Cautious volume expansion with crystalloid or whole blood
- Hypoglycaemia – Glucose administration
- Identify and eliminate precipitating event by specific treatment

8. Antithyroid drugs?

   Ans)

- Radioactive iodine (Described earlier)
- Thioamide derivatives (Dealt earlier- Along with it remember its most common side effect skin rashes and dangerous side effect agranulocytosis)
- Iodide trapping inhibitors – Thiocyanates and perchlorates (Not used)
- Thyroid hormone release inhibitors – Sodium and potassium salts of iodides, Organic iodides and Iodine (To study its mechanism remember the Wolff-Chaikoff effect studied in physiology. Increased iodine concentration paradoxically reduces the capacity of iodide trapping), Allergic reactions are its common side effects.

9. Fastest acting anti thyroid drug? Why?

   Ans) Iodine and iodides because of the presumed autoregulatory mechanism.

•••

ORAL HYPOGLYCAEMIC DRUGS

1. Classify oral hypoglycaemic drugs and explain any two groups?

   Ans)

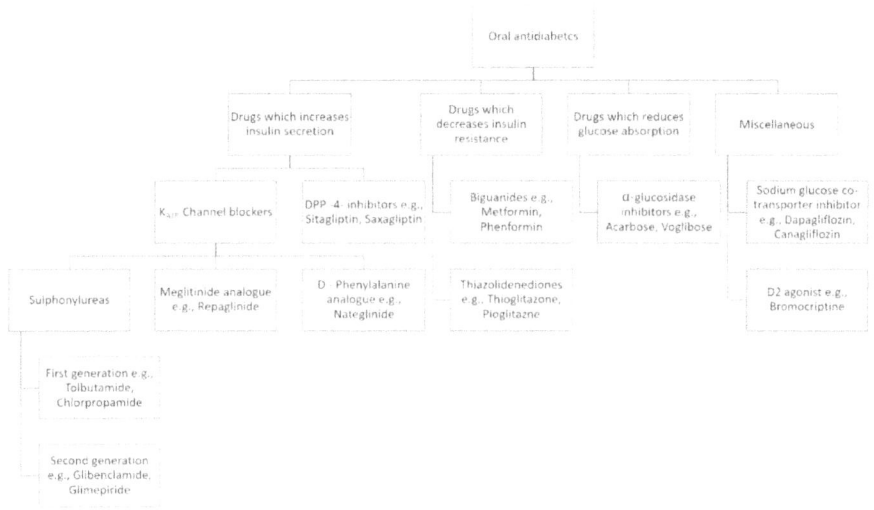

Oral hypoglycemic drugs

Examples can be studied by Thiazolidinediones includes zones, Dipeptidase – 4 -inhibitors as DIStrict, S for Sitagliptin and Saxagliptin. Alpha glucosidase inhibitor starting with A – Acarbose

Sulphonylureas

Classified into 2 generations. Second generation is more potent.
Mechanism of action

- They are insulin secretagogues they cause the release of stored insulin from the β-cells of islets of Langerhans of the pancreas by binding to the specific receptors on them and blocks the ATP sensitive potassium channels and causing depolarisation and influx of calcium ions into the β-cells which causes degranulation of the vesicles stored with insulin.
- Along with increasing insulin they also decrease the release of glucagon.
- They also increase the sensitivity of the peripheral tissues to the insulin by increasing the number of insulin receptors.

Pharmacokinetics – High oral bioavailability, High plasma protein binding and have low volume of distribution. Its metabolism happens mainly in the liver and excreted mainly through the urine.

Drug interactions – With betablockers like propranolol which blocks the symptoms of hypoglycaemia like palpitation, tremor, tachycardia also by blocking the hepatic β2 receptors it inhibits the glycogenolysis and delays recovery from the hypoglycaemia.

With Salicylates and sulphonamides which have high plasma protein binding capacity than the sulphonyl urea they displace the sulphonyl urea from the plasma proteins and increases the free plasma concentration which can cause severe hypoglycaemia

With enzyme inducers like rifampicin and phenobarbitone its effects are reduced and with microsomal enzyme inhibitors like Warfarin and Sulphonamides decreased metabolism of sulphonyl urea and can cause severe hypoglycaemia.

Adverse drug reactions – Hypoglycaemia, Weight gain, Teratogenicity, Allergic reactions

Biguanides

Metformin is the only FDA approved Biguanide available for clinical use. Another example of the group is Phenformin which is not used due tto the risk of lactic acidosis

Mechanism of action

- By activating the enzyme AMP- dependent protein kinase it decreases the hepatic gluconeogenesis and increases the peripheral utilization of the glucose in the skeletal muscle and its storage there as glycogen. It also causes the decreased lipogenesis and increased fatty acid oxidation in the skeletal muscles
- They block the alimentary absorption of glucose

Pharmacokinetics

It is having high oral bioavailability absorption happens mainly through the gastrointestinal tract and gets excreted through kidney and urine.

Uses - To treat type 2 diabetes mellitus

Adverse effects - Metallic taste, (Mnemonic – metformin -metallic taste), Weight loss, Anorexia, Skin rashes.

2. α – glucosidase inhibitors?

Ans) They are a group of oral antidiabetic drugs.

Mechanism of action – By inhibiting the α-glucosidase which helps in the absorption of carbohydrates at the brush border of the small intestine, thereby it reduces the postprandial hyperglycaemia.

Uses - To treat obese type 2 diabetes mellitus patients as it is not causing obesity as its adverse effect.

Adverse drug reactions - Flatulence, Diarrhoea and fullness.

• • •

INSULIN

1. Insulin analogues? And their advantage over conventional Insulin?

Ans) An insulin analogue is any of several types of insulin medications which are altered form of natural hormonal insulin, but still can perform the same action or modified action as human insulin.

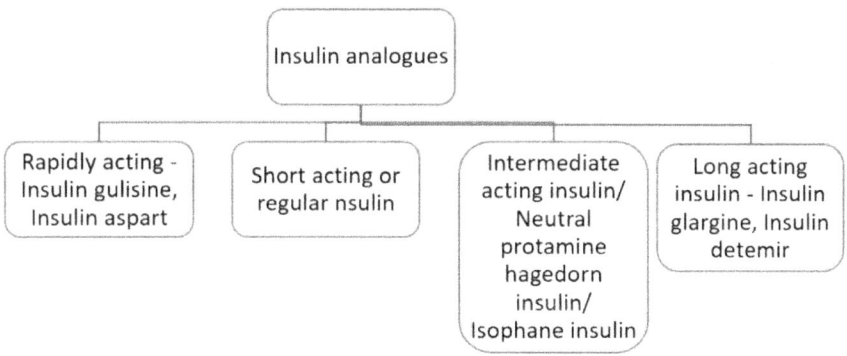

Insulin analogues

Insulin type	Onset	Peak time	Duration	Method	Examples
Rapid acting	15 minutes	1 hour	2 to 4 hours	Taken before meal	Insulin Lispro, Insulin Glargine
Regular or short acting	30 minutes	2 to 3 hours	3 to 6 hours	Taken 30 60 minutes before meal	Humulin
Intermediate acting	2 to 4 hours	4 to 12 hours	12 to 18 hours	Taken half a day or overnight	Neutral protamine Hagedorn insulin or Isophane Insulin, Lente Insulin
Long acting	2 hours	Doesn't peak	Up to 24 hours	Taken once daily	Insulin glargine, Insulin detemir

Insulin analogues properties

2. Enumerate newer insulin analogues?

   Ans)

   a. Insulin glargine
   b. Insulin detemir
   c. Insulin lispro
   d. Insulin aspart

4. Examples of anti-pseudomonal penicillin?

   Ans) Piperacillin, Carbenicillin, Ticarcillin, Mezlocillin

5. Treatment of hypertension in a patient on insulin treatment?

   Ans) Using angiotensin converting enzyme inhibitors and angiotensin receptor blockers.

6. Insulin Glargine?

Ans) It is the longest acting Insulin, given as once daily dose. It is a synthetic insulin with 2 additional arginine residues at the carboxy terminal of the carboxy terminal of B chain and glycine replaces Asparagine at the A21. Delayed onset of action, can be administered once a day, incidences of night time hypoglycaemia is less. But meal-time glycaemia is not controlled for which a rapid acting insulin or oral hypoglycaemic is used concurrently.

7. Management of Insulin resistance?

Ans) Using regular exercise and balanced diet. Drug therapy includes biguanide Metformin and Thiazolidinediones like Pioglitazone.

8. Management of diabetic ketoacidosis?

Ans)

- Short acting regular insulin 0.1 to 0.2 U/Kg iv bolus followed by 0.1 U/Kg/hr infusion.
- Rate is doubled if no improvement in 2 hrs.
- When blood sugar is reduced to 300 mg%, rate is reduced to 2-3 U/hour
- Replace fluids – 2 to 3 litres of normal saline over first 1 to 3 hours and subsequently ½ NS
- When plasma glucose level reaches 250mg%, 5% glucose in ½ NS or DNS
- KCl when plasma K^+ less than 5.5 milliequivalent per litre, guided by ECG and serum levels
- Sodium bicarbonate, phosphate if needed
- Antibiotics to treat precipitating cause

9. Two advantages of human Insulin?

Ans)

- They are absorbed more rapidly from the injection site
- Their subcutaneous injection is associated with fewer skin reactions.

10. Regular insulin or Lente insulin in the treatment of diabetic keto acidosis?

Ans) Regular insulin because of its rapid onset of action, lower hypoglycaemic risk, higher efficacy, dose can be adjusted, and highly efficacious.

...

CORTICOSTEROIDS

1. Classification of Corticosteroids?

   Ans)

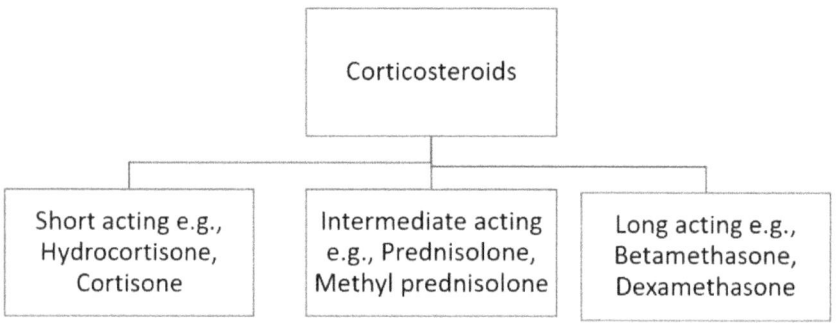

Classification of corticosteroids

2. Uses and adverse effects of corticosteroids (Prednisolone)?

   Ans) <u>Uses</u>
   It is used for the replacement therapy as well as for anti-inflammatory and immunosuppressant effects.
   <u>Replacement therapy</u>
   Replacement therapy is done to treat Chronic adrenal insufficiency, Acute adrenal insufficiency, adrenogenital syndrome and adrenal virilism.
   <u>Uses of anti-inflammatory and immunosuppressant effects</u>
   To treat

- Rheumatoid arthritis

- Osteo arthritis
- Gout
- Bronchial Asthma
- Allergies
- Eczema
- Hives

<u>Adverse effects</u>

- Cushing's habitus can occur due to increased corticosteroid
- Oedema, hyper tension can occur due to sodium water retention
- Osteoporosis and pathological fractures can occur
- Muscle weakness can occur due to hypokalaemia

<u>Contra indications</u>

- Hypersensitivity to any component of the formulation
- Concurrent administration of live or live attenuated vaccines
- Systemic fungal infections
- Osteoporosis

3. Mechanism of action of Hydrocortisone (Glucocorticoids)?

Ans) The glucocorticoids bind to the glucocorticoid receptor in the cytoplasm and form glucocorticoid receptor complex which enters the nucleus to cause its action. In the nucleus the complex upregulates the production of anti-inflammatory proteins and causes its action.

4. Inhaled corticosteroids?

Ans) Inhaled corticosteroids are medicines that contain corticosteroids such as budesonide, fluticasone. These are designed to be inhaled through the mouth and act directly in the lungs to inhibit the inflammatory process that causes conditions like asthma and chronic obstructive pulmonary disease (COPD). Because of inhaled corticosteroids deliver the medicine directly into the lungs, much smaller doses of corticosteroid are needed to effectively control symptoms compared to what would be needed if the same medication was taken orally. This also reduces the likelihood of side effects.

The persons using inhaled corticosteroids should wash their mouth well after each use to prevent the development of oral candidiasis.

5. Name two glucocorticoids with no mineralocorticoid activity?

   Ans) Betamethasone and Dexamethasone

6. DOC of cerebral edema?

   Ans) Dexamethasone and Betamethasone

• • •

GONADAL HORMONES AND RELATED DRUGS

1. Classification of hormonal contraceptives?

   Ans)

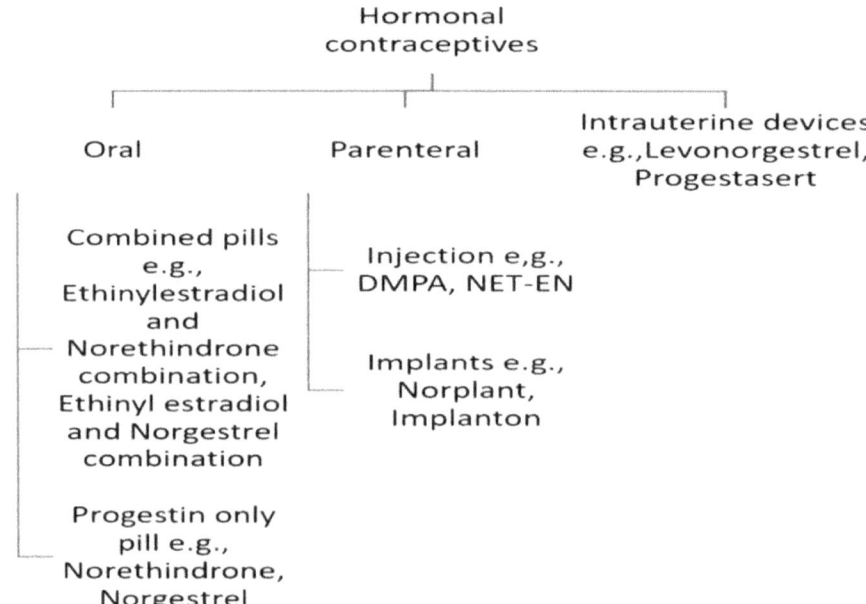

Classification of hormonal contraceptives

2. Raloxifene?

Ans) It is a selective estrogen receptor modulator. It has antiestrogenic effect in the breast and endometrium of uterus and estrogenic action on Bone, Blood and Plasma lipid.

- In the breast it stops the proliferation of ER positive breast tumours
- In the endometrium it stops the proliferation
- In the bone it reduces the resorption of bone
- In the blood it decreases the risk of venous thrombosis

Uses – To treat and prevent osteoporosis, to treat reduce the risk of ER positive breast cancer.

Adverse effects – Joint pain, Flu symptoms, Increased sweating, Leg cramps, Hot flushes, Increased incidents of deep vein thrombosis and pulmonary embolism

(Mnemonic – Tamoxifen causes endometrial proliferation whereas Raloxifene not, remember as TEacher)

3. Enumerate the advantages, disadvantages and precautions while using oral contraceptives?

Ans)

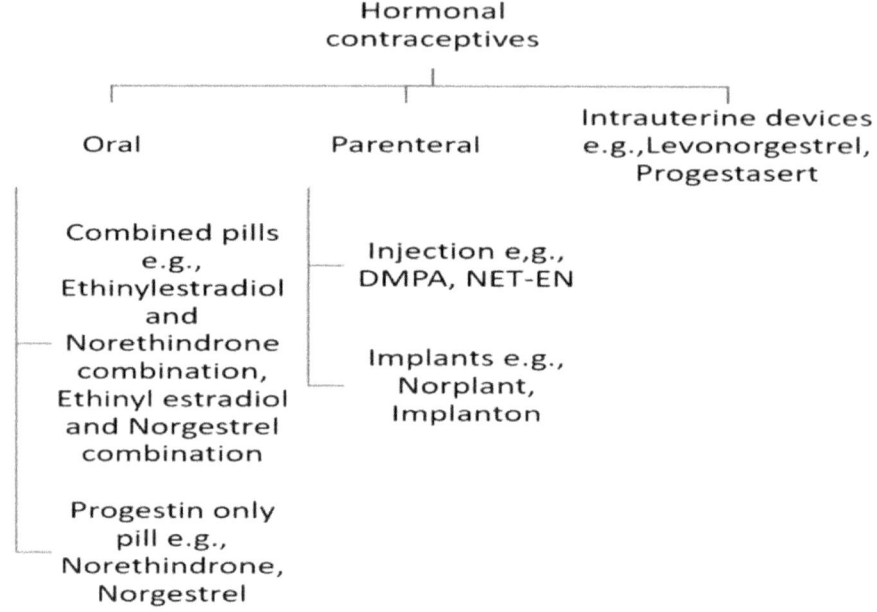

Classification of oral contraceptives

4. Clomiphene citrate?

Ans) It is a selective estrogen receptor modulator. Used to treat PCOS and female infertility

5. Anabolic steroids?

Ans) They are synthetic versions of testosterone. E.g., Dianabol, Trenbolone. Used to treat hormonal problems like delayed puberty in males and loss of muscles caused by cancer or HIV.

6. Post coital contraceptives?

Ans) Also known as emergency contraceptives. They act by preventing implantation and ovulation. They are used to prevent conception after rape, accidental rupture of condom or unprotected intercourse.

Examples – Levonorgestrel within 72 hours of unprotected intercourse
Ulipristal within 5 days of unprotected intercourse, Mifepristone 600 mg single dose

7. Mifepristone?

Ans) It is a medication which is approved for medical termination of pregnancy along with misoprostol. It acts by antagonising the action of progesterone the natural pregnancy hormone which is essential for the sustainment of pregnancy.
Adverse effects – Heavy vaginal bleeding, Severe birth defects to the child if not terminated, nausea, vomiting, diarrhoea

8. Oxytocin or Ergometrine in postpartum haemorrhage?

Ans) Oxytocin because ergometrine can cause hypertension.

9. Centchroman?

Ans) It is a synthetic nonsteroidal contraceptive with estrogen antagonistic effect.
Dose – Orally twice daily for 12 weeks and after that weekly
Pregnancy returns after 6 months of stoppage
Pharmacokinetics – Long plasma life
It has no teratogenic, carcinogenic or mutagenic effect

10. Rationale of using estrogen in hormonal contraception?

Ans) Since it prevents ovulation, Changes the uterine lining and alters cervical mucus.

11. Hormone replacement therapy?

Ans) Hormone replacement therapy is medication that contains female hormones in which the estrogen that the body stopped making after menopause in a lower level to treat menopausal symptoms.

12. Anti progestins?

Ans) Examples - Mifepristone, Ulipristal

Uses – For medical termination of pregnancy and as a postcoital contraceptive

13. Name two drugs other than oral contraceptives which will have problem when taken with phenytoin?

    Ans) Azole antifungals and some antibiotics like cotrimoxazole, Rifampicin

14. Name two gonadotropin releasing hormone agonists?

    Ans) Goserelin, Triptorelin

15. Prolactin inhibitors?

    Ans) Bromocriptine, Cabergoline

• • •

DRUGS ON CALCIUM BALANCE

1. Bisphosphonates?

   Ans) It is a class of drugs which decreases bone resorption.

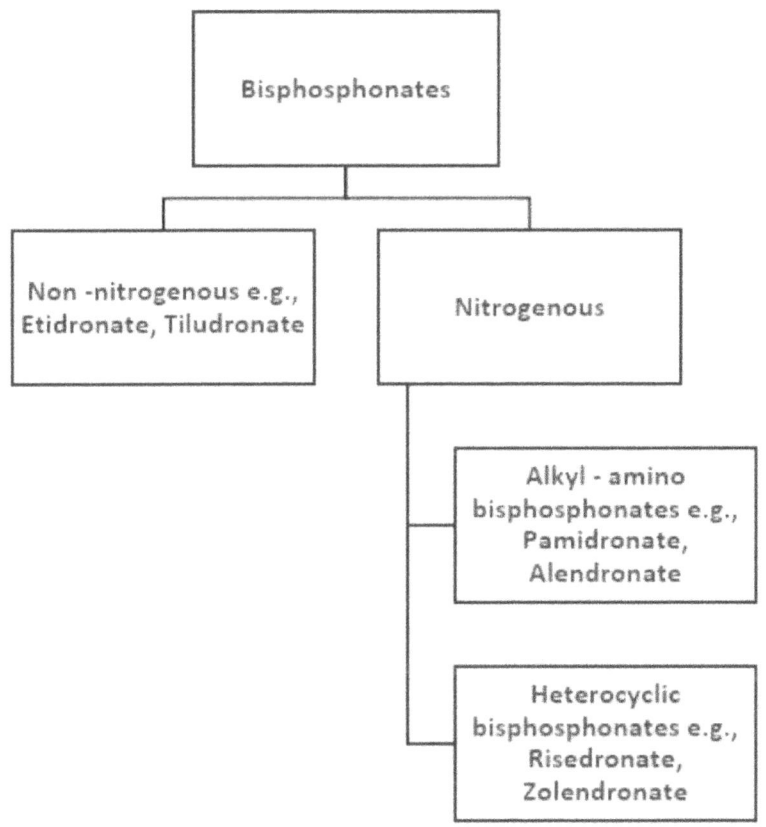

Classification of bisphosphonates

Examples – Tiludronate, Pamidronate, Alendronate, Zoledronate and Etidronate.

Mnemonic – They are drugs which decreases the PAZE of bone resorption.

Mechanism of action

- Having high affinity with calcium in the bone it accumulates in areas with high bone resorption and is taken up by the osteoclasts and they inhibit the ability of the osteoclasts to form ruffled border and causes their apoptosis

- They interfere with the cholesterol synthesis pathway which is required for the proper function of osteoclasts.

Pharmacokinetics - Poor oral bioavailability but those which are absorbed will remain in bone for longer time as months to years. Excretion happens through kidneys.

Uses

- To treat Paget disease of bone
- To treat post-menopausal and corticosteroid induced osteoporosis
- To treat hypercalcaemia in pregnancies, hyper parathyroidism
- To relieve pain of lytic bone lesions

Adverse effects – Hypocalcaemia, Myalgia, Peptic ulcer, Skin rashes

CHAPTER XIII

Miscellaneous

IMMUNO SUPPRESSANTS

1. Cyclosporine?

   Ans) It is an immunosuppressant drug of class Calcineurin inhibitors
   Mechanism of action – It enters the target cells and binds to the intracellular protein cyclophilin and forms cyclosporine-cyclophilin complex and prevents formation of calcineurin as cyclophilin is required for calcineurin formation.
   As calcineurin is required for the activation of T cells they are not activated and the production of IL-2 and other cytokines are reduced and causes reduction of cell mediated immunity.
   Uses – To prevent graft rejection & to treat autoimmune disorders like myasthenia gravis, systemic lupus erythematosus, rheumatoid arthritis etc.
   Adverse effects – Hepatotoxicity, Nephrotoxicity, Hyper lipidaemia, Hyper glycaemia, Hyper trophy of gums, Hirsutism and due to the decreased immunity infections increases.

2. Tacrolimus?

   Ans) It is an immunosuppressant drug of class Calcineurin inhibitors.
   Mechanism of action – Same as cyclosporin except the binding protein is different.
   Uses and adverse effects are also same as cyclosporine

3. What immunosuppressant drugs are required to inhibit rejection of transplant?

   Ans) Cyclosporine, Tacrolimus, Everolimus, Azathioprine, Sirolimus and glucocorticoids are used. Sirolimus is preferred over cyclosporine in renal failure patients because sirolimus does not acts via the calcineurin pathway and doesnot produce the same renal side effects.

4. Immunotherapy for Rh negative woman with Rh positive baby?

Ans) Anti Rh immunoglobulin (RhoGAM) is given as soon as the delivery is over.

• • •

Drugs acting on skin and mucous membrane

1. Calcipotriol?

Ans) It is a synthetic form of calcitriol (Vitamin D3) which is used to treat psoriasis

2. Psoriasis drugs with their pharmacological basis of usage?

Ans) Vitamin D – Since deficiency of it can plaques cause the keratinocytes to proliferate and lead to the development of thick, scaly plaques which are a common symptom of psoriasis.
Corticosteroids – It can reduce the redness, swelling, scaling and itch.

3. Anti-seborrheic agents?

Ans) Selenium sulphide and zinc pyrithione

• • •

Chelating agents

1. Penicillamine?

Ans) It is a chelating agent used to treat copper poisoning, lead poisoning, zinc poisoning and mercury poisoning. Since it promotes the excretion of copper in case of Wilsons disease it is used to treat it, lifelong therapy is required. Other diseases treated with It (Mnemonic - Screen the other diseases), S – Scleroderma, C – Cystinuria and R -Rheumatoid arthritis.

Adverse effects – (the SP's PUPiL) S – Scleroderma, P- Pruritus, PL- Pemphigoid lesions.

2. Desferrioxamine?

Ans) It is a chelating agent which can be used to chelate iron. It causes separation of iron from the ferritin and hemosiderin at the same time not from the haemoglobin, also affinity to calcium is low so the chances of deficiency of calcium in the blood is low.

Uses – To treat chronic iron poisoning as seen in thalassemia intramuscularly whereas to treat acute iron poisoning Desferrioxamine is given intravenously other uses are to remove the aluminium during dialysis.

Adverse effects - Allergy, Flushing, Rashes, Itching (Mnemonic – AFRI)

3. Oral iron formulations and its adverse effects?

Ans) Ferrous sulphate, Ferrous fumarate and ferrous gluconate
ADR – Abscess and discolouration at the site, Urticaria, Arthralgia, Lymphadenopathy.

• • •

ANTISEPTICS AND DISINFECTANTS

1. Antiseptics?

Ans) Antiseptics are chemicals which can be applied to the skin that stops or slowdown the growth of microorganisms e.g., Chlorhexidine and povidone iodine.

• • •

ANTICANCER DRUGS

1. Methotrexate?

Ans) Methotrexate is a cell cycle specific anti-cancer drug which blocks the cell cycle at the S-Phase of the cell cycle. As we have studied in our NCERT textbooks S-Phase is the synthesis phase where the synthesis of DNA takes place. For the synthesis of DNA Tetrahydro folic acid is essential (THFA) by competitively blocking the dihydrofolate reductase it prevents the formation of tetrahydro folic acid.

Uses – To treat choriocarcinoma, (Mnemonics – Meth Kori (Scratched in the body), Burkitt lymphoma, Breast cancer, Acute leukaemia

Uses other than for cancer – Low dose methotrexate is used to treat rheumatoid arthritis, psoriasis, inflammatory bowel disease and organ transplantation due to its anti-inflammatory and immunosuppressant effects.

Drug interactions – Salicylates, Tetracyclines and sulphonamides which can displace methotrexate from plasma proteins can cause its toxicity.

Adverse effects – Hepatic fibrosis, Pancytopenia and Megaloblastic anaemia.

Folinic acid rescue or Leucovorin rescue – As any other anticancer drug when we use high doses the drug it will cause damage to the surrounding normal cells also. But in case of folinic acid can reverse the toxic effects if given after getting required effect so that high doses of the drug can be given which is called as Leucovorin rescue or folinic acid rescue.

2. Thalidomide?

Ans) Thalidomide was olden days prescribed for morning sickness of pregnant women, which caused the birth of so many babies with congenital defects like phocomelia, and there by banned it. Now it is using in the treatment of Lepra reaction.

3. Vinka alkaloids?

Ans) Vinka alkaloids they are cell cycle specific anti-cancer drugs which are blocking the cell cycle at the M-Phase, obtained from plants. Examples, Vinblastine and Vincristine.

Mechanism of action – They causes no formation of intact microtubules by binding to the β tubules and preventing its polymerisation.

Vinblastine – In case of use starts with B, breast cancer which is one cancer predominant in females and in males' testicular cancer and causes adverse effect bone marrow suppression.

Vincristine – Uses starts with c, Child hood tumours like Neuroblastoma and Wilms tumour, Child hood leukaemia's and Hodgkin disease. Adverse drug reactions peripheral neuritis.

4. Taxanes?

Ans) Taxanes are a Cell cycle specific anti-cancer drugs.

For example, Paclitaxel and Docetaxel

Mechanism of action – As it is cell cycle specific it blocks the cell division at the metaphase of the cell cycle by leading to the formation of abnormal microtubules by stabilizing the microtubules by binding to its monomer β tubulin (Whereas in Vinka alkaloids NO microtubules)

Mnemonics – Since we are paying taxes, they will make something but not good. Taxanes – abnormal microtubules

Uses – To treat lung cancer, bladder cancer, breast cancer ovarian cancer etc.

Adverse drug reactions – Myalgia, bone marrow suppression peripheral neuropathy and hypersensitivity reaction.

Other cell cycles specific drugs – Anti metabolites, Antibiotics, Vinca alkaloids, Epipodophyllo toxins, Taxane (Mnemonic –reached at **vet** in a cycle) here t in at represents 2 groups in starting with A

5. Cyclophosphamide?

Ans) It is a cell cycle non-specific anticancer drug of the class alkylating agents and among it under nitro-gen mustards.

Mechanism of action – Being a prodrug it reaches the liver get activated into phosphoramide mustard and acrolein among it the phosphoramide have the tissue toxic effect and is responsible for its anticancer effect, whereas acrolein causes haemorrhagic cystitis.

Pharmacokinetics – Well absorbed orally, excreted through kidney

Uses – To treat malignancies like Chronic lymphocytic leukaemia, breast cancers, lymphomas etc, also to treat autoimmune disorders like rheumatoid arthritis, graft rejection during organ transplantation and nephrotic syndrome.

Adverse drug reactions – Due to the acrolein haemorrhagic cystitis can occur which can be decreased by co-administration of MESNA intravenously. Bone marrow suppression, Alopecia and Hyperuricaemia are also seen

6. Letrozole in breast cancer?

Ans) Letrozole being an Aromatase inhibitor inhibits the production of estrogen in the body. Since the ER positive breast cancers require estrogen to grow it is used to treat ER positive breast cancers.

7. Rationale for the use of combination of drugs in cancer chemotherapy?

Ans) The rationale is tumor cell heterogenicity and its implication for drug resistance and the success of combination chemotherapy in the clinic

8. Anti-malignancy drugs producing gouty arthritis?

Ans) Paclitaxel and gemcitabine.

CHAPTER XIV

Assertion and Reason questions

A - If A & R are true and R is the correct reason for A
B - If A & R are true but R is not the correct reason for A
C - If A is correct and R is incorrect
D - If A & R are incorrect

1. A - Levocetrizine is preferred over Chlorpheniramine maleate for rhinitis in a machine operator

    R - Levocetrizine doesnot causes sedation
    Ans) A (A & R are true and B is the correct reason for A)

2. A - Adrenaline is preferred in Anaphylactic shock

    R - Adrenaline is a chemical antagonist against Histamine
    Ans) C - Adrenaline is a physiological antagonist against Histamine

3. A - Digoxin acts by inhibiting the sodium potassium ATPase

    R - Digoxin can cause ventricular tachy cardia
    Ans) B

4. - A - Atorvastatin is used in dyslipidemia

    R - Atorvastatin is H+, K+ ATPase inhibitor
    Ans) C (Atorvastatin is a HMGCOAreductase inhibitor)

5. A - Bioavailability is 100% with intravenous administration

    R - Drugs given intravenously directly reach systemic circulation
    Ans) A

6. A - Sildenafil is used to treat erectile dysfunction and pulmonary artery hypertension

B - It inhibits the phosphodiesterase-3 enzyme
Ans) C (Sildenafil inhibits phosphodiesterase-5- enzyme)

7. A - The antibacterial action of Dapsone is antagonized by PABA

   R - The mechanism of action of Dapsone is by incorporating the PABA into the folic acid by folate synthase
   Ans) A

www.ingramcontent.com/pod-product-compliance
Lightning Source LLC
Chambersburg PA
CBHW050257230526
45471CB00005B/1925